RELIGIOU[S]
IN YOGA

Lectures on Theory and Practice

T.K.V. Desikachar

Edited by
Mary Louise Skelton
John Ross Carter

UNIVERSITY PRESS OF AMERICA

LANHAM • NEW YORK • LONDON

University Press of America,™ Inc.

4720 Boston Way
Lanham, MD 20706

3 Henrietta Street
London WC2E 8LU England

Printed in the United States of America

ISBN (Perfect): 0-8191-0967-3
ISBN (Cloth): 0-8191-0966-5
LCN: 79-9643

All University Press of America books are produced on acid-free paper which exceeds the minimum standards set by the National Historical Publications and Records Commission.

TO MOTHER

Srimati Namagiriammal

FOREWORD

Religiousness in Yoga by Mr. T. K. V. Desikachar is the result of a course offered during a January Special Studies Program at Colgate University, 1976. For a number of years, Colgate University has been conducting a program during the month of January in which undergraduates take only one course of study. In some cases, faculty members design courses that might be of special interest to undergraduates at a particular time. In other cases, faculty members develop courses at the "cutting edge" of their own research and invite students to share this study with them. Occasionally, specialized projects and programs are instituted for students that might be difficult to execute during an ordinary semester. And, on occasion, a concentrated series of readings, a period of study and practice is designed for maximum teaching and learning effectiveness in a context that enables a student to maintain sustained concentration and reflection unobstructed by other course requirements.

Reflecting all of these cases, a January Special Studies Program, "Religiousness in Yoga," was conceived by us and was offered in the Department of Philosophy and Religion at Colgate. We invited Mr. T. K. V. Desikachar, Managing Trustee and Teacher at the Krishnamacharya Yoga Mandiram in Madras, India, to provide lectures on some of the ideas embodied in the tradition of yoga and guidance in the discipline of postures and related practices.

The classes were attended by thirty undergraduates, three women from Hamilton, and two Colgate professors. Classes were held in the chapel of Chapel House to assist the students quickly to discern and long to remember that yoga has been nurtured by an impressive religious tradition; that the subject to be understood adequately is to be understood comprehensively, that yoga has engendered qualities of religiousness not unfamiliar to persons living in the West, qualities of religiousness as persons living in India have long known them.

The thirty-five participants were on different levels of initial competence in yoga and consequently four sections were organized. Those who had some experience comprised two groups that met on each week day for one hour of instruction in postures and in breathing procedures. One-hour sessions for instruction in postures and breathing techniques were held three times a week for the two groups of beginners. Every afternoon all participants met for lectures by and discussions with Mr. Desikachar. Three afternoons each week, these lectures were on the principles and purposes of yoga and twice each week, on alternating days, there were discussions related to the practice of yoga with special reference to the postures and breathing techniques. These lectures and discussions are now presented in this volume.

This book does not represent a comprehensive treatise on yoga, nor is it an argument seeking, by marshalling evidence, to persuade a reader, nor an attempt to "convert" a reader. Rather, this book is a result of an act of sharing a religious undertaking, an act of sharing now appearing in printed form.

In transcribing the recorded lectures and through the editing of the drafts, we have made every effort to keep the structure as it developed in the sequence of the January course. We hope that the reader will sense a "live situation" in order more readily to become engaged with the subject. The questions appearing in the book are authentic and were transcribed from the recordings of the lectures. They have received only minor editorial revision.

We wish to express our appreciation to Mr. T. V. Anantanarayanan for his drawings utilized in this book. Mr. Gary Kraftsow, a participant in the January Program, a student of Mr. Desikachar, gave generously of his time in Madras, 1977, in helping during the initial stages of editing. We are grateful to Professor William Skelton, Chairman, Department of Music, Colgate University, for his thorough reading of the manuscript and his valuable suggestions. Mrs. Elizabeth H. Davey, Secretary to the Director of Chapel House, demonstrated unusual perseverance in checking the manuscript during its various stages of development. Mrs. Patricia Ryan patiently produced the typed form of the final manuscript.

Our special thanks are due to the American Institute of Indian Studies for their generous support of Mary Louise Skelton in Madras, during the summer of 1977, to continue her work in yoga and to begin the editing with Mr. Desikachar. We acknowledge our appreciation to the Colgate University Research Council for a grant to assist in our editorial work in Madras. The Fund for the Study of the Great Religions of the World, Colgate University, sponsored the January Special Studies Program, "Religiousness in Yoga," and continued financial support for our work on this project throughout the editorial process in India and in the United States.

Mary Louise Skelton
Instructor in Yoga

John Ross Carter
Associate Professor of
Philosophy and Religion
Director, Chapel House

Hamilton, New York

PREFACE

When I conducted the course "Religiousness in Yoga" at Colgate University, I had no idea that what might transpire would be considered for publication. During that month of January, 1976, the students, other participants, and I gradually developed a mutual relationship of learning and the result of such a phenomenon is difficult to express. These lectures and discussions, printed words put before persons I might never meet, are but reflections of that deeper result that grew out of a living face-to-face encounter. Coming to learn of yoga only through reading leaves much to be desired. Yet, something worthwhile about yoga might be shared through the medium of the printed word.

Too numerous to list here are those to whom I wish to express my gratitude for their enthusiastic support for a book like this one. Especially, I wish to thank my students, who have taught me very much. In agreeing to the publication of these lectures and discussions, I am following the sound judgment of my colleague Mary Louise Skelton and Dr. John Ross Carter and here wish to thank them for their work in editing the several drafts and in seeing the final manuscript through publication.

To my teacher and father, T. Krishnamacharya, who has taught me and guided me into what I know, I salute.

T. K. V. Desikachar

Krishnamacharya Yoga Mandiram
Madras, India

SANSKRIT PRONUNCIATION GUIDE

Vowels:

a	as in	hut
ā	as in	father
ī	as in	beet
i	as in	hit
u	as in	put
ū	as in	pool
ṛ	as in	"er" (with a trill of the tongue and a slight "i" off-glide)
ṝ	as in	ṛ but lengthened, somewhat like reed
ḷ	as in	"el" (with a trill of the tongue and a slight "i" off-glide)
e	as in	bed
ai	as in	isle
o	as in	tow
au	as in	out

Consonants:

k	as in	kite
kh	as in	book-house
g	as in	goat
gh	as in	dog-house
ṅ	as in	sing
c	like "ch" in cheese	
ch	aspirated as in coach-horse	
j	as in	just
jh	like "dgeh" in hedgehog	
ñ	somewhat like ñ in señor	
ṭ	as in	treat
ṭh	as in	rot-house
ḍ	as in	rod
ḍh	as in	road-house
ṇ	as in	spring
t	as in	toe
th	as in	boat-house
d	as in	doll
dh	as in	hid-her

n	as in	no
p	as in	pat
ph	as in	up<u>h</u>old
b	as in	bath
bh	as in	ab<u>h</u>or
m	as in	me

<u>Semivowels</u> (voiced):

y	as in	yes
r	as in	rich
l	as in	long
v	as in	view (but a gentle fricative, almost an English "w")

<u>Sibilants</u> (unvoiced):

ś	as in	sugar
ṣ	as in	sweet
s	as in	see

Visarga	ḥ	a light voiceless aspirate
Anusvāra	ṃ	a nasal lengthening of preceding vowel

TABLE OF CONTENTS

I

Theory

THE MEANING AND PURPOSE OF YOGA

Today I will share with you some reflections about the meaning of yoga. Yoga is one of the six principle systems of Indian thinking known as *darśana*. The word *darśana* is derived from the Sanskrit root *drś*, meaning "to see." Fundamentally, *darśana* means "view" or "a particular way of viewing." It also has a further meaning which suggests a mirror, a mirror in which we might see ourselves. Yoga, as one of the six *darśana*, has its source in the *Vedas*. The word *veda* comes from the Sanskrit root *vid*, "to know." It means "that which tells us everything we would like to know." While the source of yoga was the *Vedas*, this particular *darśana*, yoga, was formalized by Patañjali, one of the great Indian sages. His classic text is the *Yoga Sūtra*. Although there are many other major treatises on yoga that postdate Patañjali's *Yoga Sūtra*, his work is the most authoritative.

What is yoga? So much has been written and said about yoga that you must forgive me if I repeat some basics you might already know. The word "yoga" is also a Sanskrit word derived from the root *yuj*. *Yuj* has developed two traditional meanings. One is "to bring two things together, to meet, to unite." For example, before these lectures I was in Madras. I did not know where you were before this meeting but now we are together. The other meaning is similar to that of *samādhi*, that is, "to converge the movement of the mind." Although these definitions might appear different, they are really the same. Our being here together represents the *yuj-yoga* concept of yoga. At the same time, our converging paths from our various homes to Hamilton, New York, then Colgate University and finally to this chapel at Chapel House represents the *yuj-samādhi* concept of yoga. We have gone in the same direction; we have converged; therefore, we are together.

Another meaning might be of greater importance as well as more engaging. That meaning is "to reach a point we have not reached before." If there is something that is impossible for us to do today and we find a means by which it becomes possible, that movement is yoga. In fact, any movement such as finding a means by which we can flex the body in order to touch our toes, or learning the meaning of the word yoga through a text, or the understanding that comes through dialogue; any of these movements is yoga. We have reached a point where we have not been before.

Another important aspect of yoga has to do with action. Yoga also means "to act in a particular way with all of our attention focused upon that action." Suppose that while I am speaking to you about yoga one part of my mind is thinking about what I will say while another part thinks of something else. As I become more involved in lecturing, my attention to my action of speaking increases. I am focusing upon my actions. Sometimes it is the opposite, when I begin an action I am very attentive but as I proceed my attention wavers. This is the result of man's great facility to develop habitual processes and patterns of thought and behavior. We become conditioned. We appear to be acting with attention but there is no attention. We are functioning but we are not present. Yoga tries to create a condition in which we are always present in every action, at every moment. When we begin to do <u>āsanas</u> (postures) together, we will see how these concepts can be introduced into our physical practices.

The advantage of attention to action is that we act better, and at the same time we are conscious of our actions. Our chances of making errors will be less and less as our attention increases. Further, we don't have to do something today just because we did it yesterday. If there is attention to our actions, there is always a chance for us to reassess them and especially to avoid mindless repetition.

Yet another classic definition of yoga is "to be one with the Lord." No matter what name we use--Īśvara, God, or Allah--any movement that makes us understand something higher than ourselves is also yoga. Being one with the Lord means we understand and respect something that is higher than what we understood yesterday. When something within us feels in tune with something higher, that too is yoga.

With so many definitions available, it is important to remember that the practice of yoga calls for direction. This direction does not require specific movements or predetermined ends. It does require us to watch cautiously the direction of each step we take in order that we know exactly how and where we are going. These cautious observations will lead to discovery. Whether this discovery leads to a better understanding of the Lord, or more contentment with life, or another goal is a personal matter.

Who should practice yoga? Is it necessary to hold certain beliefs in order to follow the path of yoga?

The practice of yoga only requires that we act and at the same time, pay attention to our actions. We do not have to endorse any particular concept of the Lord, but we must have respect for such concepts. Although yoga has its source in Indian thought, it neither dictates that a Hindu must practice it nor that a non-Hindu is prohibited from such practice. Yoga is universal in that it is the means to attain a desired new condition. If we want to be happier and we find the means to that happiness, that is yoga. I'm sure that this is not uniquely Indian but universal in its appeal.

Where and how do we begin the practice of yoga? Should it always be physical?

How we begin depends upon our individual interests. There are many ways to practice yoga. Gradually, the practice of one technique will lead to others. We might begin by studying the Yoga Sūtra, or we might begin with prayer. We might begin with āsana so that, through bodily feeling, we understand yoga. We might begin with breathing; feeling the breath as inward movement. There are no restrictions as to where and how we begin our practice.

There are no required or special disciplines.

It is often suggested, in texts and through personal instruction, that there are preconditions to the study of yoga; that we must discipline ourselves in order to begin the practice of yoga. We are told that we must not smoke; that we must be vegetarians; that we must give up all worldly goods; that we must follow some model. Such suggestions are unfortunate. While these actions may be admirable, they occur within us as the effects of yoga, not as causes. For example, people have told me that they were habitual smokers prior to their practice of yoga. They began yoga and, as a result of their work, they no longer wanted to smoke. They did not stop smoking in order to practice yoga. We begin where we are, as we are, and what happens, happens.

There is another important point about our practice. When we begin the study of yoga either through _āsanas_, _prāṇāyāma_ (disciplined techniques of breathing), prayer or the _Yoga Sūtra_ we are dealing with but one technique of learning. As we progress, we notice that we are whole beings consisting of body, breath, mind, and more. Some persons, who begin their practice with _āsanas_, persist in learning more and more postures until, to them, the sole meaning of yoga becomes physical exercise. This is like a man who develops only one beautiful, strong arm while allowing the other to remain weak. Similarly, there are people who only intellectualize the concept of yoga. They write wonderful books, they speak magnificently about _prakṛti_ and _ātman_ but can't sit straight for a few minutes in order to write or talk. So please remember, we might begin the practice of yoga at any point but, as complete human beings, we must gradually look at all aspects of ourselves. In the _Yoga Sūtra_ we see the emphasis placed upon all aspects of human life, including such things as our relationships to others, our own behavior, our health, our breath, and our _dhyāna_ (meditation).

Why should one practice yoga?

I doubt that there is anyone who doesn't really want

to be better. "I am poor, I want to be rich." "I am confused, I want to be less confused." "I want to study engineering." "I want to become qualified in medicine." What are all of these but the desire to be better? These desires to be better are served by yoga. Through the practice of yoga we gradually improve our capacity to concentrate, our self-reliance, our health, our relationships--in fact, all that we do.

Having briefly mentioned the source of yoga--what yoga means, who can practice it, and why we should practice it--I would like now to consider a very important concept drawn from Patañjali's Yoga Sūtra. It is a concept which, if understood properly, explains why we have problems in life. If we know why we have such problems we will know how to get rid of them. This is the important concept, avidyā. Avidyā means literally "knowledge other than right knowledge." It is not to be confused with vidyā which means "right knowledge." Avidyā is a false state of understanding. We think we are right and we act accordingly but eventually we find ourselves on the wrong track. Equally troublesome, we may have an understanding that we think is wrong which in fact is not. Therefore, we don't act when we should. What is this avidyā embedded within us?

Avidyā is the accumulation of actions. It is a culmination of many thoughtless actions that we have repeated mechanically, almost blindly, over the years. Our minds become so conditioned that we accept yesterday's actions as today's norms. Such conditioning is called saṃskāra. Because of this conditioning our minds become covered, as it were, with a film of avidyā.

Avidyā often does not express itself as avidyā. If we know that we don't understand and we are sure of that, we will not act and if we know that we understand, we will act and we will be right. This action is based upon a deep level of perception. Quite the opposite, avidyā expresses itself through superficial perception that says, "I think I know, then I act, and find out later that I didn't know." We go wrong because we think we know, when in truth, we don't; or the reverse, we think we don't know, when in truth, we do. Therefore, we have two levels of perception. One is deep within us and is free of the film of avidyā. The other is superficial and is covered with avidyā.

This concept of avidyā explains much that happens in life. For example, at Chapel House where we can find silence and solitude, it would be difficult for avidyā to expand. Little by little, avidyā subsides and truth is revealed. Then we see clearly how we should act. This is the goal of yoga, that we reduce the film of avidyā in order that we can act correctly.

How is avidyā expressed?

Avidyā rarely expresses itself as avidyā. We seldom experience it immediately and directly; however, we will know it through its four children. First is asmitā. It is the "I thing" which is always pushing us. "I should beat him." "I am the greatest." "I know I am right." "I can't fail"--all of these are expressions of asmitā. Second is rāga which is attachment or desire. We want something today because it was pleasurable yesterday, not because we need it. Yesterday we had a piece of cake that was delicious. Today something in us says we wish we had another piece of the cake even though we don't need it. Third is dveṣa, in some ways the opposite but with the reverse effects of rāga. If we don't get what we want, we tend to hate it or we have a bad experience and we don't want it to happen again. Finally there is abhiniveśa, which is the source of fear. This is the most mysterious aspect of avidyā. No matter what its source, abhiniveśa has ramifications at many levels of our daily existence. We feel insecure. We have fears about our position in life. We dread how others judge us and those close to us. We feel insecure when the continuity of our way of life is disturbed. We don't want to face old age. All of these are rooted in abhiniveśa, the fourth child of avidyā. These four children, separately or in combination, make it difficult for us to see clearly.

Avidyā is constantly working behind us and is the source of much discontent. It is often very difficult to understand our distress at one moment and our happiness at another. As an example, in a group session practicing *āsanas* there is the inclination for us to compare ourselves with others. We think, "Oh, he can bend his body more than I can," and this brings unhappiness. But the practice of *āsanas* is not a competitive athletic event. Just because one person can bend more than another does not prove or disprove that the former is better in the practice of yoga. Such comparisons cannot be the basis of happiness or unhappiness. They may lead us to a happiness based upon superiority, or the opposite, unhappiness over inferiority. Often this unhappiness is so severe that it makes us quit our pursuits. giving up in despair.

Let me give another example of the persistence of *avidyā*. In the course of a conversation with a friend, I make a mistake. Usually, I will feel quite humble and apologetic. Yet at another time, with the same friend, I might be discussing the *Yoga Sūtra*. He might say that I am speaking nonsense and my interpretations of this great text are wrong. Do you know what my reaction might be? Something deep inside me aches. I am unhappy. How can I react this way? Do I try to prove my friend wrong? Should I try to escape from the situation? In this example we see how the mind works. We fear we are losing ground. We show hatred because yesterday's satisfaction over a pleasant event may not help in today's different situation.

Finally, as long as the children of *avidyā* are in the ascendency, there will always be the chance that we can go wrong since careful discretion and thorough discrimination will be absent. What yoga does is to reduce the action of *avidyā*, in order that true understanding prevails.

Question: Is *avidyā* present when we are born or is it something we acquire as we grow older?

Response: There are two views. Let's consider them in the context of fear, one of the four children. One view is that the only fear that really matters is the fear of death. We have not died and yet we have the fear of death. Thus, we must have experienced death in a previous life and the bitter memory of death is born with us. The other view is that fear can develop during our lifetime. I remember the first time my son climbed a ladder. He had no fear until he slipped and fell. The second time he climbed, he cried, "Hold it, hold it, hold it"--meaning the ladder. While I cannot positively say that his fear developed because of his fall rather than the fear from a previous birth, I feel quite sure that many of our actions during our present lifetime are enough to give us such fears. The Yoga Sūtra says that even the wisest man has fear. How can this be? He has fear because he has made mistakes during this life and because of these mistakes he has become cautious. This caution is the beginning of fear. Caution, in small amounts, can be good but sometimes too much caution keeps us from functioning.

Question: You said that avidyā does not express itself directly as avidyā and that yoga is the reduction of avidyā. Do we have to become conscious or aware of avidyā in ourselves in order to reduce it? How can we reduce it if it doesn't express itself?

Response: The reduction of avidyā is seen through the reduction of its effects. When there is less asmitā, rāga, dveṣa, and abhiniveśa, then there must be less avidyā. We notice avidyā by its absence, not by its presence. When we recognize previous troubles we know that avidyā has been present.

Question: You said earlier that sometimes we think we are right and sometimes we think we are wrong but vidyā is knowing we are right, that is, we see things clearly. What is the distinction of avidyā when we think we are right and vidyā when we know we are right? Does our mind just know? Is it intuitive?

Response: These are good questions because they reveal a special trap. When we know we are right, there is deep within us a feeling of quietness; no tension, no disturbances, no excitement. When I speak slowly, deliberately, I know there is a source of quietness, and there is vidyā in me. However, when I am not sure of what I am saying, I tend to speak quickly, I use unnecessary words, and I break my sentences. When our understanding is clear, we feel something serene deep within us. There is no disturbance.

There are several other concepts I would like to introduce. According to yoga, everything we see, experience, and feel is not an illusion but true and real. This concept is called sat-vāda. Everything, including avidyā, dreams, and even fancy and imagination, is real; however, all these things are constantly in a state of flux. This concept of change is called pariṇāma-vāda. The way we see things today might not be the way we saw them yesterday because those things, our relationship with those things, and we ourselves, change. In yoga although everything we see and experience is true and real, changes do occur either in character or in content. It is because of this concept of change that we do not have to worry about avidyā. If things are going poorly, they can always change for the better. Of course things can also take a turn for the worse. We never know what might happen in life, so we must be careful. Whether things get better or worse is to quite an extent in our hands. That is why the practice of yoga, called sādhana, is suggested. Sādhana is the means by which we reach a previously unattainable point.

However, there is in the concept of yoga something deep within each of us that is real and not subject to change. We call it draṣṭṛ or puruṣa. It is what sees and can see correctly. The practice of yoga is to let this happen. As long as the mind is covered by avidyā, our observations are clouded. When we feel deep within us a quietness and we understand something, such an understanding is what matters and it will have a strong positive influence. However, this true understanding which occurs as the result of the reduction of avidyā generally does not happen spontaneously. This complex of body and mind has become accustomed to particular patterns that tend to change very gradually. In any case, change from confusion to clarity should be gradual in order to avoid shock. In the Yoga Sūtra it is said that in the beginning of one's sādhana, clarity and confusion follow each other in cycles, like a wave-form. That means we have some clarity, alternating with confusion.

As we progress there will be less and less confusion and more and more clarity.

Question: Is that which is deepest in me, my *puruṣa*, different from every other *puruṣa*?

Response: The word *puruṣa* means "the person who resides in the city." *Puru* means "city, town, township." The one who stays in the town is the *puruṣa*. What is the nature of this town? It consists of the body, the mind, the senses, our culture, customs and even *avidyā*. If we eliminate the town, all *puruṣas* are absolutely the same, but they appear different since they reside in different towns.

Question: Doesn't a conscious decision to engage in the practice of yoga demand a recognition of *avidyā*? Is it not an expression of *asmitā* to want to be better?

Response: These questions may lead us to important discoveries about the purpose of *avidyā*. We have *avidyā* and when we recognize that, directly or indirectly, we realize we must do something about it. While our first step, namely "I want to be better" may be rooted in *asmitā* or ego, it is the right step because it is on the first rung of the yoga ladder. Further, we are not permanently committed to this early concept of betterment. According to the *Yoga Sūtra* recognition and elimination of *avidyā* and its effects is the only ladder we can climb. To aim for something better may be the first rung of the ladder. If we can start above the first rung, namely "I want to be better," we probably don't need yoga.

How can we make this climb?

Again I refer to Patañjali's *Yoga Sūtra*. Three things are suggested by which we can begin to explore the meaning of yoga and therefore feel *avidyā*. First is *tapas*. *Tapas* comes from the root word *tap*, "to heat, to cleanse." *Tapas* is a means by which we keep ourselves fit and clean. Often *tapas* is defined as penance, mortification, and dietary austerity, but what is meant here is the practice of *āsana* and *prāṇāyāma*. Apart from other benefits, these

KRIYA YOGA - YOGA OF ACTION

practices aid us in the removal of impurities from our system. In so doing we gain control of our whole system. It is the same principle as heating gold to purify it.

The next means by which we can explore yoga is svādhyāya, the study of ourselves. Where are we? What are we? What is our relationship to the world? Sva means "self." Adhyāya means "study." It is not enough to keep ourselves fit. We should know who we are and how we relate to others. This is not easy because we don't have an actual mirror for our own minds as we do for our bodies. We must resort to reading, study, discussion, and reflection as a mirror to the mind. This is especially true with the great works such as the Yoga Sūtra, the Bible, the Mahābhārata, and the Qur'an. Through the study of such texts we "see" ourselves. ingiry

The third means of exploration as suggested in the Yoga Sūtra is Īśvara-praṇidhāna. It is usually defined as "love of god" but it also means "quality of action." Practicing yoga āsanas and prāṇāyāma, keeping fit, and reading scriptures do not constitute our only actions. We must also carry out our jobs, go to college; in fact, do everything expected of us. All of these actions must be done with a high degree of quality. Since we can never be certain of the fruits of our labors, it is better to remain slightly detached from them and pay more attention to the actions themselves. quality of action

Together, these three (tapas, svādhyāya, and Īśvara-praṇidhāna) cover the whole of human action: fitness, inquiry, and quality of action. If we are fit, know more about ourselves and improve the quality of our actions, chances are we will make fewer mistakes. These are three specific practices that are recommended to reduce avidyā. Taken together, these practices are known as kriyā yoga, the yoga of action. Kriyā comes from the root word kṛ, "to do." Yoga is not passive. We must be involved in life, and preparation is necessary for this involvement.

Finally, and to repeat, there are two aspects of yoga: yoga as action; yoga as result. At the beginning of this lecture I suggested that yoga is that state in which two things have been brought together as a completed act. I also suggested that yoga is attention to actions necessary to reach a heretofore unattainable position or point. The means by which we obtain the yoga of result is the yoga of action, kriyā yoga. While only part of yoga, kriyā yoga is the practical aspect of yoga which can initiate a change for the better in the quality of our lives.

II

Practice

THE PRINCIPLES OF PRACTICE

The practice of yoga provides us an occasion that might give us a feeling for the meaning of the word yoga. Despite any incidental benefits, this is the fundamental reason for practice. In the first session we defined yoga as a movement from one point to a higher point. Whether this movement occurs in posture or in mind it is yoga. It is also yoga if it brings insight about the highest truth.

In our practice we focus upon the body, the breath, and the mind. We include the senses as part of the mind. While it is theoretically possible for the body, the breath, and the mind to work independently, it is the purpose of yoga to unify their movement. In our very first practice classes, we will experience this unification. What appears as yoga to an outsider is mainly the physical aspects of our practice. They will not be aware of how we breathe, how we feel the breath, and how we coordinate breathing with physical movement. They tend to be interested only in our flexibility and suppleness. They count our postures. They time our headstands. What is more important, however, is the way we feel our breath and posture. Longstanding principles, developed by generations of teachers, guide us in yoga practice. These principles detail posture and breathing, especially as they relate to each other. In addition, they define the whole course of our yoga practice. They also establish guidelines for prāṇāyāma. These will be described later.

What is an āsana? Āsana means "posture" and it comes from the Sanskrit root, ās, "to stay, to be, to sit, to be established in a particular position." Patañjali's Yoga Sūtra describes āsana as having two important qualities: sukha and sthira. Sukha is the ability to remain comfortably in a posture. Sthira is firmness and alertness. Both qualities should be present in a posture. It is neither sukha nor sthira for us to sit cross-legged while being photographed and then have to immediately straighten our legs. Even if we achieve sthira, firmness and alertness, it must also involve sukha, time and comfort. Without both qualities it is not an āsana. Therefore, if we practice a particular posture over a period of time, being at ease, alert and comfortable, then the principles of practice are fulfilled.

All of the following principles are designed to make sure that each āsana is both sukha and sthira. If we are doing an activity in which we are tense, we cannot observe anything but our tension. Suppose we sit in a cross-legged posture and our only thoughts are about the pain of our ankles pressing together. We are not completely in the posture, nor are we ready for that particular posture. We must do something simpler. This is the idea behind our whole technique of practice. As we progressively do postures, we very gradually have more sthira together with more sukha.

To make this idea of an āsana a reality, we must accept ourselves as we are. Therefore, if we have a stiff back, we must acknowledge that fact. Perhaps we are very supple but our breath is quite short; perhaps our breath is all right but our body isn't ready, then we cannot have the qualities of āsana. It is also possible to be very comfortable in a posture while our minds are elsewhere. This, too, is not āsana. We will later see that if the breath does not go uniformly with the movement of the body there is something wrong. The quality of breath is very vital since it expresses our inner feelings. If there is pain it shows itself through the breath. Though we can facially mask our pain through training, we cannot control our breath during pain. If there is distraction we lose control of the breath. The breath is the link between the inner and outer parts of our bodies. This is why the body, the breath, and the mental movement must merge in order to have the qualities of āsana.

The first step toward recognition of our total condition is called svādhyāya. It begins with self inquiry into our physical condition, including our breathing. To begin, we use simple dynamic movements involving the arms, legs, and trunk. This morning in a beginners' class, you were asked to raise and lower your arms. It was a very simple movement. You were then asked, "Did the arm movement stretch your back or some other part of the body?" Some of you said that the movement stretched the back. Others said they felt stretching in the shoulders. This means one of two things: either the same movement was done differently or some of you have stiff backs and all of the work went to your shoulders. You can see how important it is to make this kind of investigation of our own bodies; however, at the beginning a teacher is necessary to guide you through these discoveries. In a group class, if a teacher is unable to follow the unique conditions of each student, it would be unfortunate, since not only would we not understand yoga, we might also be discouraged.

The next step is to investigate our breath. Take a deep breath and try to make the inhalation as long as possible. In this way, we will see whether the chest or the abdomen expands, and whether the back stretches with the breath. As we raise our arms, inhale. As we lower our arms, exhale. This is the first level of yoga practice, the merging of the breath and the body. In order for the breath to work with the body, our minds must be attentive to the process because of conscious inhalation-exhalation. This is not an automatic process. Normally, we are not conscious of our breathing. In order to merge the breathing with the movement, the length of our inhalations and exhalations determines how fast our arms are raised or lowered. In this first movement of raising the arms on inhalation and lowering the arms on exhalation, we will understand a fundamental dimension of yoga which is to be totally involved in our action.

It doesn't matter how beautifully we do a posture or how flexible our bodies are, if we do not have the unification of the body, the breath, and the mind, it is difficult to say that our practice falls within the definition of yoga. After all, what is yoga? It is something we experience inside, within our whole being. It is not an external experience. Even a blind or deaf person doing a posture can feel and discover yoga.

Let us examine, step by step, the principles involved in this practice. The most important principle is the natural relationship between breathing and movement. We will see that the body has a particular relationship to the breath. As in any physical activity when we squeeze the body, pressure forces the breath out. We breathe out in all postures where bending is in a particular direction, such as a forward bend of the back.

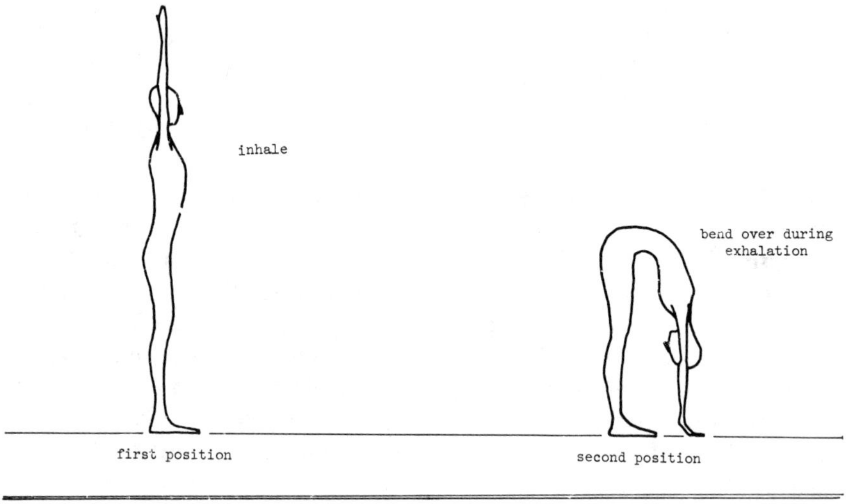

Fig. 1

We inhale when we reverse the direction.

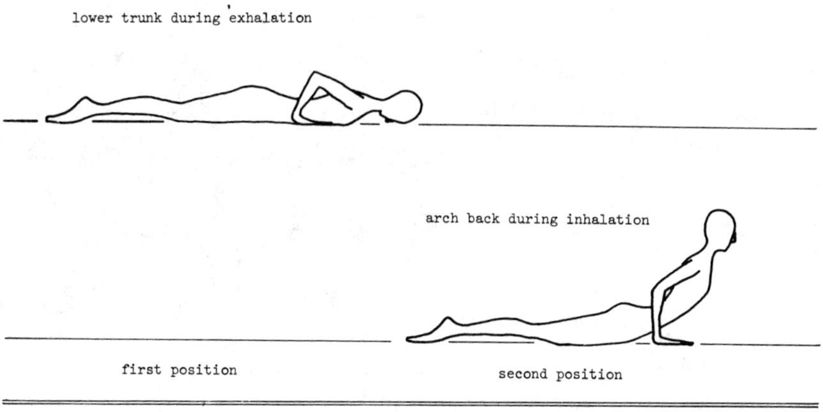

Fig. 2

Similarly, whenever we raise our arms overhead, we inhale and when we bring them down, we exhale.

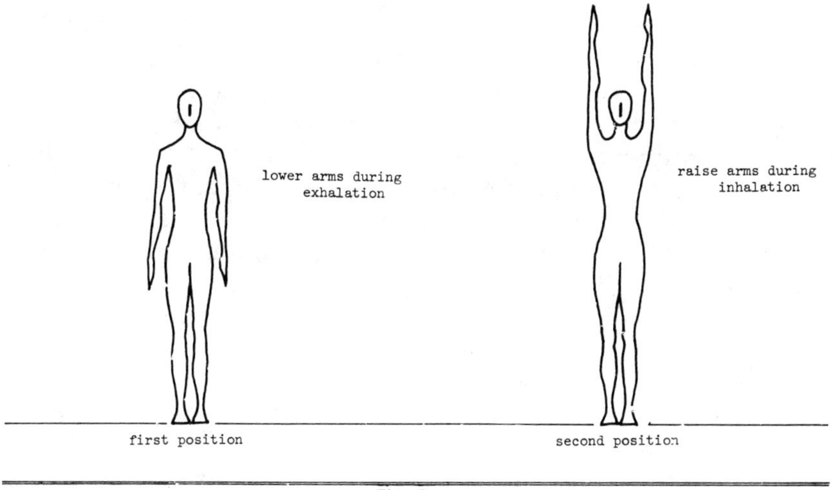

Fig. 3

This type of coordination establishes the relationship between breathing and movement. One more movement of the body affects breathing. This is torsion or twisting. Any torsional movement of the body calls for an exhalation. When the body untwists, we inhale.

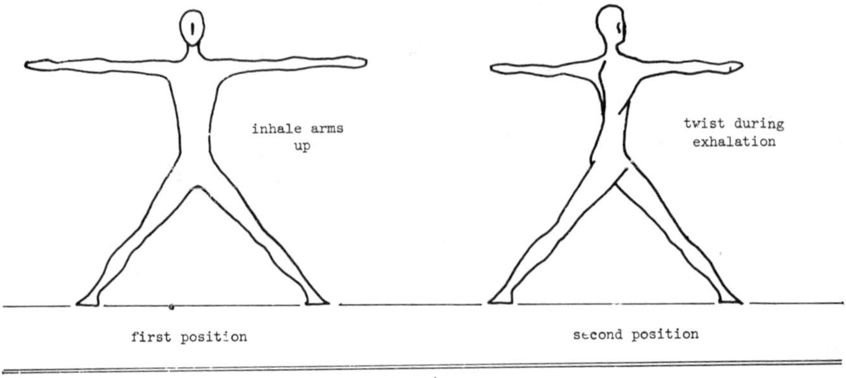

Fig. 4

These rules are very simple--when we contract the body, we exhale; when we expand the body, we inhale. At the same time, we are not simply inhaling and exhaling, we are making sure that the breathing and movement go together. This comes only through practice. If we take four seconds to raise our arms and six seconds to lower them, we must inhale four seconds and exhale for six. So first, we determine the length of time for our inhalations and for exhalations. This fixes the timings of our movements. Merging of the breath and movement will become almost automatic as we practice.

We have mentioned briefly the conditioning processes of our mind and how we can develop habits so quickly. To avoid this habit forming tendency, we always introduce a small break or gap at the end of each movement. For example, after we raise our arms on inhalation, we hold for one or two seconds. When we lower our arms on exhalation, we again hold for one or two seconds. This must be done so that deep within us, we are always in control of our breath. Without control our actions are done out of habit. We break habit formation by these rules.

What is the technique of breathing? We use a particular technique that involves total, deeper breathing under conscious control. Deep inhalations expand the chest and move the diaphragm downward. This expansion of the chest and abdomen is required for us to inhale. When we exhale, we do the opposite. We contract the abdomen on exhalation and as we do this, the ribs contract. This is the technique

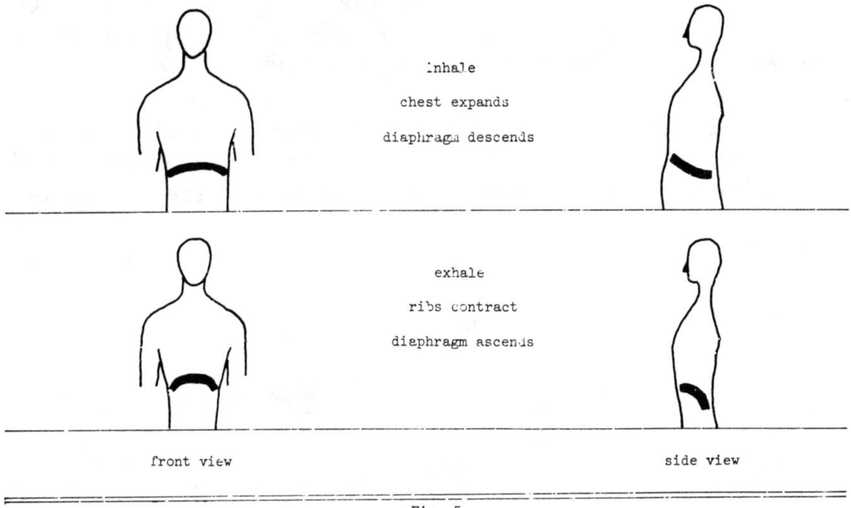

Fig. 5

we try to use. Often people breathe solely with their abdomens with no expansion of the chest. Others cannot use the diaphragm because of too much weight or because they are too tense. Tense people and asthmatics can hardly use the chest or abdomen. In such cases we must use different breathing techniques. Ideally, our technique is to expand the chest and abdomen on inhalation, and contract the abdomen on exhalation. This technique of breathing is another means of bringing quality to our practice of yoga. We now have a coordination between breathing and movement as well as a particular technique of breathing.

Our next step allows us to feel the breath throughout inhalation and exhalation. Through this we will gradually improve the quality of our technique of breathing. This technique is also conscious and not automatic. If we breathe through the nostrils quickly, we create a sound but no feeling of quality about the breath. This is true whether we are breathing uniformly or not. To give us this feeling of uniformity and smoothness when we breathe, we impose a restriction on the throat which produces a sound. It is as if we had a valve in the throat and we partially closed it to control the breath. We measure the control by the sound. This sound is produced uniformly during both inhalation and exhalation, allowing us to hear, as well as feel, the breath as we work toward deeper and longer cycles.

There are two advantages to using this technique. One, we are more involved with the flow of the breath, and therefore, we have concentration throughout the <u>āsana</u>. Two,

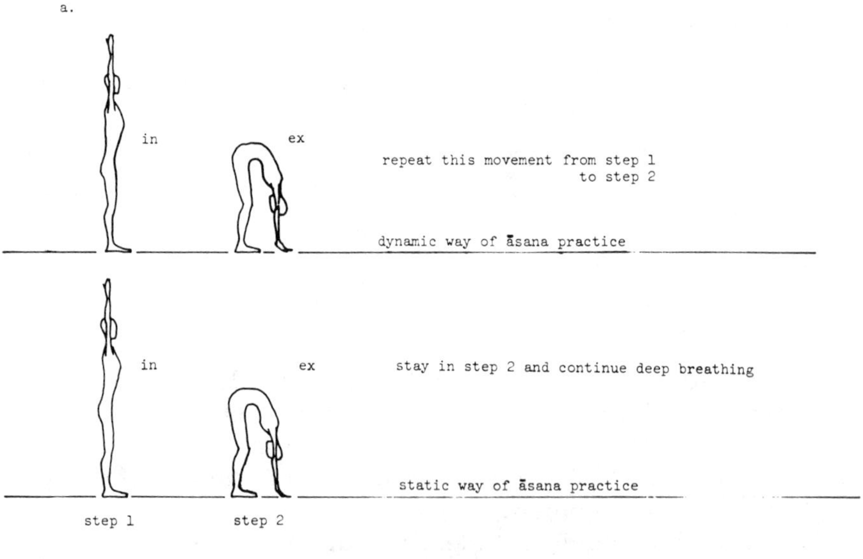

Fig. 6

Breath determines limits

the sound in our throats tells us when to stop or change an āsana. We do āsanas in two ways--dynamic and static. In beginning practice, we do āsanas in the dynamic way. We bend over, touch the floor and immediately come up. This is the only possibility for the beginner since, if they are asked to stay any length of time they might develop problems. Dynamic movements lead to the second phase, static postures. This in turn leads to longer and longer periods of firmness and alertness in postures (sthira). Beginners often have the problem of not knowing how many times to do a posture. For example, if they are asked to stand, bend over and touch their toes and come up a total of twelve times, how can they know whether twelve is the proper number of times? Legs might tire, the effort might be too much or they might feel back pain, though pain is not always immediate in overexertion. None of these symptoms are good indicators of our limits. Only the breath will determine this. As long as we can breathe smoothly with the sound in our throat, we are within the limits of our body. The moment we need to take a quick breath through the nostrils without maintaining the proper throat sound, we must stop. Obviously, these principles of practice will not be introduced on the first day since the practice of yoga is very gradual.

Another concept of breathing used during our practice is called "holding the breath." After we inhale, we hold the breath and at the same time stop all movement. Similarly, after we exhale, we also hold the breath and stop all movement before our next inhalation. As with inhalation and exhalation, holding the breath is a conscious act. The length of time we hold the breath is critical. If it is too long, either after inhalation or exhalation, the body rebels. Now, how is this practice introduced? When we hold the breath in posture, it must never disturb inhalation or exhalation. For example, while doing a posture we might inhale five seconds and exhale five seconds comfortably. When asked to hold the breath five seconds after inhalation, we find that we need a quick breath. This means we are not ready for this technique. If the holding of the breath is too demanding, the inhalation and exhalation will be disturbed. Holding the breath should be practiced only as an aid to inhalation and exhalation. Some of us might be able to inhale five seconds and exhale ten seconds with or without holding the breath. For us, this technique is recommended. However, if we hold our breath after inhalation and it shortens our exhalation, or if we hold our breath after exhalation and our inhalation becomes short, we are either not ready for holding the breath or we are trying to hold too long. The first reaction of the body when we hold too long is to demand a quick breath. Without it, our bodies will tremble. When investigating holding of the breath, please remember that we must not disturb our inhalation or exhalation.

It seems there are innumerable āsanas and just as many books published about them. These books compete to see which can list the most postures. One text describes eighty-four postures, another lists two hundred, and so-called definitive books on yoga list even more. Such lists are endless because the great flexibility of the body allows almost unlimited variations of postures. Some postures are so difficult, they cannot be photographically recorded. Whether it is worthwhile doing many or few postures depends upon the individual. Different people need different āsanas. Some of us, especially myself, are so stiff-legged, that we need to stress standing postures. Others such as dancers with flexible, well-formed legs may be so supple that there is no need for them to emphasize standing postures. While there are many postures, we do not have to do all of them. We must plan a course of practice that meets our own needs, and through which we can discover the qualities of āsana. At the same time we must prepare ourselves for other aspects of yoga such as sitting comfortably and doing deep breathing.

We will now examine some of the basic āsanas and the principles that apply to these postures. If we can understand the principles of simple postures, we will have no difficulty practicing the more difficult ones. In the beginning stages of daily practice, we need to do some postures through which we can observe the condition of our breath and body. We are different every day. If we have eaten heavy food the night before, we will be stiff. If we didn't sleep well, we might have a headache. Legs are often stiff for no apparent reason. Climatic conditions also influence the body. For example, January in upstate New York is so cold that I need to stretch my back before sitting on the floor.

What postures should we choose? Postures to make us limber are needed and the best of these are the standing ones. Standing postures are designed to loosen all moving joints, such as ankles, knees, hips, spine, shoulders, neck, and to some extent the wrists. Obviously, elderly people with leg problems or people with other difficulties might not be able to begin with standing postures; however, most of us should limber up with standing postures for five to ten minutes.

We have postures that counter the great effect that gravity plays in the function of our bodies. Gravitational effects are both good and bad. Yoga tries to undo the latter. As an example, among the bad effects of gravity are a curved spine, stooped shoulders, neck thrust forward and organs pulled downward. We try to reduce the negative effects of gravity by using the body in a different plane. This is achieved through inverted postures. To accomplish this, there are supine postures where we simply lift the legs and, of course, the headstand and the shoulderstand which are the complete opposite of normal posture. The effect of gravity also affects the muscles. When we are uncomfortable sitting in a slumped position, it is not that gravity has an increased effect upon us, it is because the muscles of our backs are unable to take the unusual loads. Also, if we are unable to sit straight, our breathing is inhibited. Therefore, we need prone postures to strengthen back muscles in order that they can resist the forces of gravity.

Finally, sitting postures help us to sit comfortably on the floor or in a chair so that we can do some breathing exercises.

The following is the usual order of our practice:

Practice Sequence

Standing
Supine
Inverted
Prone
Sitting, Kneeling
Rest
Breathing

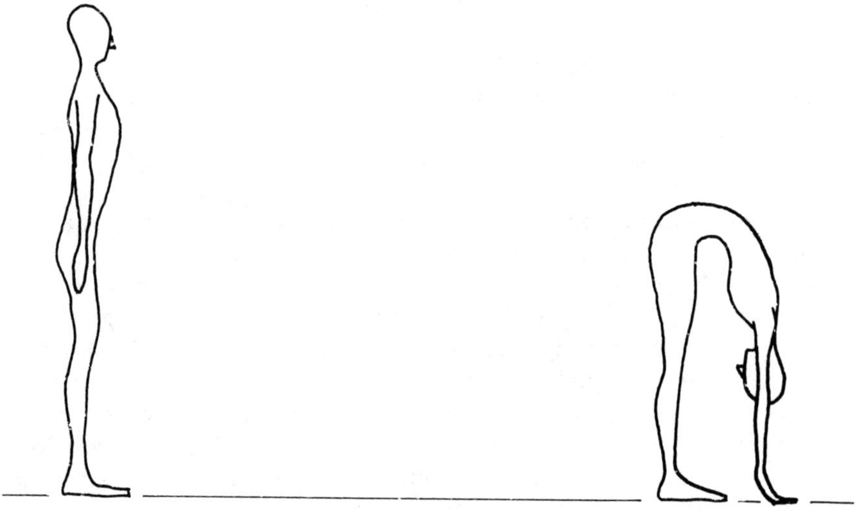

standing

Fig. 7

supine

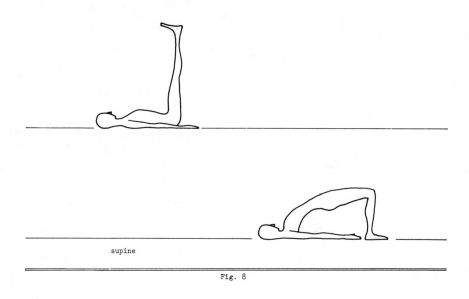

Fig. 8

inverted postures

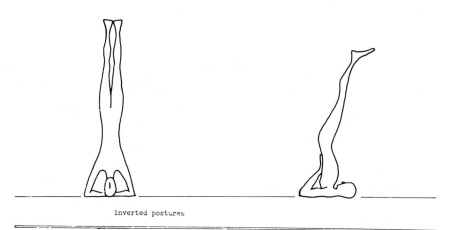

Fig. 9

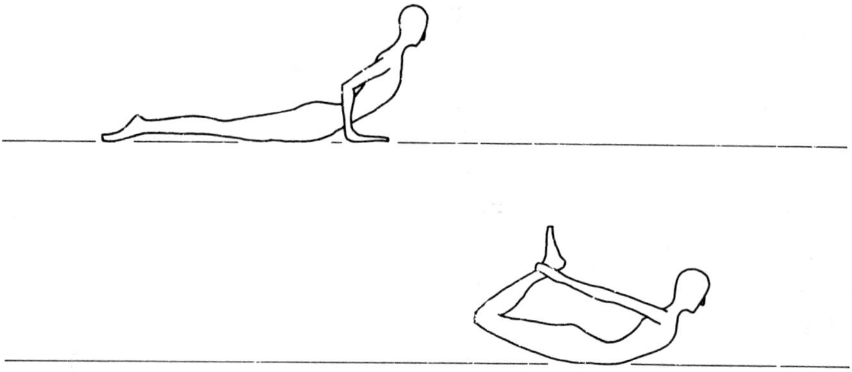

prone postures

Fig. 10

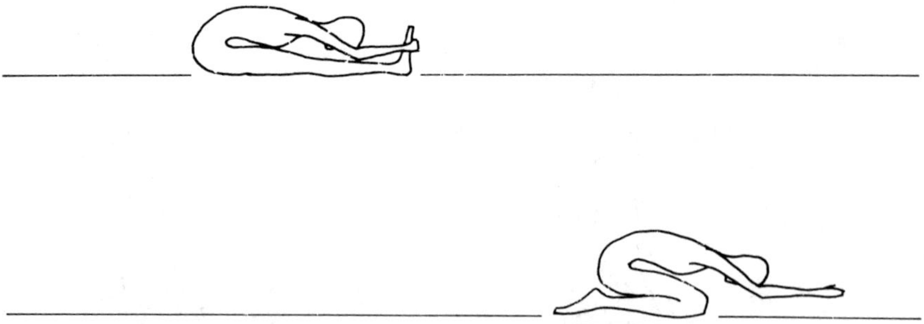

seated posture

kneeling posture

Fig. 11

rest

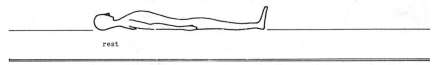

Fig. 12

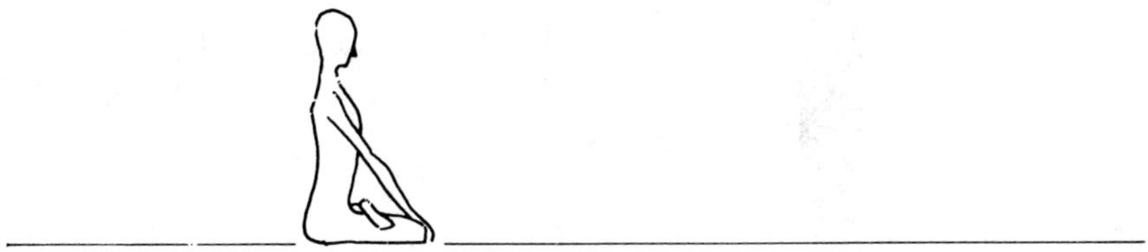

breathing

Fig. 13

Our plans must consider two other aspects of yoga practice. First, yoga teaches us that with every action there is both a positive and negative effect. While it is good for me to lecture because it helps me communicate, after two hours of speaking my throat is tired, a negative effect. Anything we do in life will have both a positive and a negative effect. This is why attention to our actions is so very important. We must recognize what effects are positive and what effects are negative. Then we must stress the positive while we neutralize the negative. In all details of <u>āsana</u>, we must follow this principle. Take the headstand as an example, some say that they can't get through a day without doing the headstand. They will do a ten-minute headstand first thing in the morning or before they go to bed at night. They feel a great sense of well-being. They do no preparation, they just stand on their heads. What they do not recognize is the negative aspect of the headstand. While the headstand is usually good, in that it reverses the customary effects of gravity on the body, it also places all the weight of the body on the neck. Our small necks, created to carry only the head, must now carry most of the body. Therefore, after a

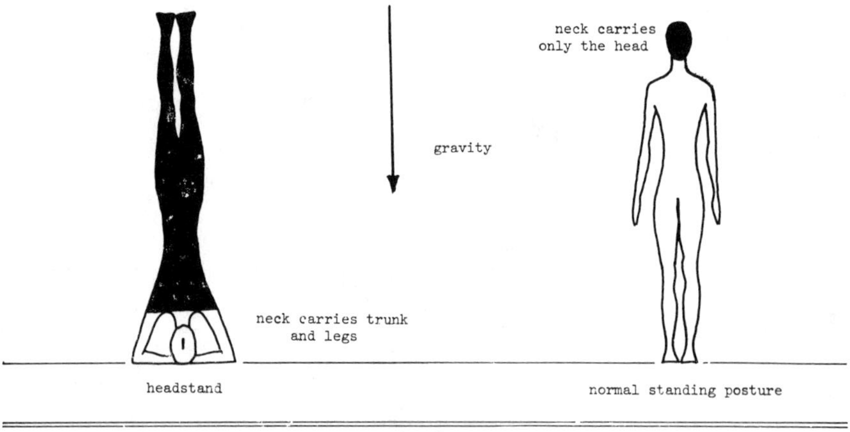

Fig. 14

headstand we must neutralize this negative aspect by doing a counterpose. If we don't, our necks will become stiff. In no time, we might even feel numbness in our fingers because of the compression of the vertebra on the nerves.

The second most important aspect is preparation. Before we do a posture we should be sure our bodies are ready for it. If we try to sit cross-legged the first thing in the morning, and we have not observed our bodies or prepared our legs, we might hurt our knees. If we prepare well, there is less need for a counterpose. But counterposes are required with some postures such as headstand, shoulderstand, bending backward, and twisting. Later I will discuss preparation and counterpose in detail. Are there any questions on <u>āsana</u>, the technique of breathing, how to coordinate the breathing and movement, the holding of the breath and the practice sequence for an <u>āsana</u> course?

<u>Question</u>: When we inhale, you said we use first the chest and then the diaphragm or abdomen and that the exhalation is the opposite. In studying voice I was taught the other way.

<u>Response</u>: Abdomen to chest; I know.

<u>Question</u>: Would you please comment on the difference?

<u>Response</u>: This is a usual question because many teachers of music train their students to breathe first from the diaphragm and then the chest. They often use the analogy of filling a bucket with water, pointing out the impossibility of filling the top first. The technique we shall use not only gives us a little more concentration, but it also stretches the spine and arches the back. The moment we inhale, our ribs expand and stretch the spine to which they are attached. With this kind of breathing, the spine is not only stretched upward, but it becomes straighter. When we use the diaphragm to chest breathing technique, the abdomen expands so much that it inhibits the expansion of the chest, and the spine is not stretched. Also with this diaphragm movement, the lower abdominal organs are pushed down-

ward. This diaphragm to chest technique of breathing, while useful in some fields, is of little value to us. We are concerned with breathing that is compatible with movement and the stretching of the spine. Please experiment with both of these methods and you will feel the difference.

Question: I have been doing exercises in another discipline and I have been told to concentrate on the center of my being, in the diaphragm area. I was wondering if there is a separate part of the body that you concentrate on, such as the forehead or throat. And if so, is that where you put all of your attention?

Response: Attention must be where there is maximum action--because then the action will be much more profound. When we inhale, for example, our action moves from the chest to the navel; when we exhale, the action is centered in the abdomen. Also, there is secondary movement on inhalation when the lower abdomen comes forward. Therefore, when we inhale our attention is on the chest and diaphragm, and when we exhale, our attention is on the abdomen. This, then, is a form of meditation if we are completely involved in the action and nothing else. This is the same attention to action we discussed earlier. A person adept at this may focus upon any zone of activity.

III

Theory

THE CONCEPTS OF AVIDYĀ AND DUḤKHA

Before continuing, let me briefly review some of the points covered in the first lecture. The source of yoga is the Vedas. Some of the many definitions of yoga are: to move from one point to another point; to bring two things together; to act with continuous attention to that action. On the basis of these definitions, starting points need not be the same for everybody, nor the same each day. Also, the point we reach need not be the same. Though there are many possible definitions of yoga, all must incorporate movement. This movement must be to a point we have not previously reached. That is to say, what was impossible becomes possible, what was not reached can be reached, what was not seen can be seen. In this context yoga means both the action by which two things meet and the result of that meeting. Yoga means both movement and result.

I mentioned that yoga has been systematized by Patañjali in his Yoga Sūtra and that it is the most authoritative text on yoga, although there are many other major treatises. I then discussed why one should be involved in yoga, who should be involved, whether there are any preconditions, or other such concerns. The reasons to be involved in yoga are to better oneself; to think more clearly, to feel better, and in all things to be better today than yesterday. There are no preconditions or prerequisite beliefs necessary to begin yoga. Further, our own religious beliefs will not interfere. Because yoga has its origin in India, one need not be a Hindu to practice it. Also, the practice of yoga is not required of the Hindu. Anyone can start. Our starting points will be as different and personal as each of us.

I suggested why we need this movement from one point to a better point. We cannot always be our best or see things clearly because we have in us an inherent cover that the *Yoga Sūtra* calls *avidyā*. This concept of *avidyā* is an understanding that might be right or wrong; however, we do not recognize which it is. Action that is done when there is *avidyā* could be wrong and therefore have negative results. Thus *avidyā* affects our actions.

I also explained that in the yoga point of view, everything is real and there is no illusion--there is no *no*. Even *avidyā*, which is the source of many problems, is valid and real. All that we see and experience is accepted. This concept is called *sat-vāda*. But all these things are in a state of flux. How we see things today may not be the way they appear tomorrow. This concept is called *pariṇāma-vāda*. Beyond that which we see and experience is what is called *puruṣa* which is the seer. It does not undergo any change but even its perception is clouded by the film of *avidyā* covering the mind.

I also explained how *avidyā* expresses itself in four forms. One way is *asmitā*, the feeling of I. I know, I am right, I can't be wrong. Another is *rāga*, the desire to have things whether we need them or not. Another is *dveṣa*. When things go badly, we dislike them. Finally and worst of all, is fear, *abhiniveśa*. Somehow we don't want to lose something. We are afraid to die, as though we had already experienced death. These are the four ways *avidyā* expresses itself. The practice of yoga is designed to reduce *avidyā* so that there is more and more true understanding. How will we ever know when we have understood or seen things clearly? We know this when something deep within us is very serene and quiet. When we see the truth, when we reach a point that is higher than ourselves, there is a deep satisfaction. It is not the emotional satisfaction we get from looking at a beautiful object, but a satisfaction deep within us that is without emotion or sentiment.

The center of this satisfaction is called *puruṣa*, "the person who stays in the city." Each of us has a *puruṣa* and this *puruṣa* appears differently in each of us because it resides "in a different city." As our conditioning is different our *puruṣa* appears to be different.

Question: You spoke of Īśvara-praṇidhāna and action with detachment. In that context would you please define detachment?

Response: I said that yoga is both movement to and arrival at a point. The yoga that we practice, the yoga in which we can progress and the process of this movement, is called kriyā yoga. The Yoga Sūtra defines kriyā yoga as having three components. Tapas, not mortification or penance, is something we do to keep ourselves fit physically and mentally. We keep ourselves clean. We remove things that we don't need. This is followed by svādhyāya. Gradually we must find out where we are, who we are, what we are, etc. This is where we begin our āsanas. We start by examining our breath and body. Hopefully this will lead us to a further understanding of our basic condition so that we will know where to begin. Concerning Īśvara-praṇidhāna, the literal meaning is "prostrating love towards God." Īśvara means God; praṇidhāna means prostration. In kriyā yoga, Īśvara-praṇidhāna need not be taken as love toward God because the acceptance of God is optional in yoga. That is, we don't have to accept a notion of God to understand yoga. The meaning given to Īśvara-praṇidhāna in the context of kriyā yoga then is a particular attention to our acts. When we act, we emphasize the quality of action, not so much the fruit of such action. Before we act we set the goals for our actions. By the time we complete the actions, we might not need these goals. If we must make a million dollars and we work toward this goal for two or three years, during that time we might well discover that our goal is unnecessary and that we should work toward something else. To maintain a flexibility in action in order to respond to our improved clarity, we must act with detachment toward the fruits of our actions. Also, if we concentrate upon process rather than goals, we avoid the disappointment of not reaching our goals. That is the meaning of Īśvara-praṇidhāna in kriyā yoga.

Question: When we were talking about āsanas, sukha and sthira were mentioned. Did you say that sthira is being aware of what we are doing but sukha is a sort of detachment?

Response: Yes, in a way you are right. If a posture, whether dynamic or static, is not comfortable, that is, if we do not feel sukha, we are not in a condition to be good observers. If there is an absence of sukha, that is, if we force ourselves into a posture, it is not a true āsana. Sukha is a state of mind where we are so comfortable that we can observe ourselves. Suppose we are agitated by onlookers as we work. We cannot have sukha because agitation blocks out our concentration. If I am physically near you, and at the same time detached, your presence is inconsequential. This is the concept of sukha, to be at ease. To be at ease does not mean to be a dullard. It means to be alert and relaxed, therefore, able to see things clearly. Sthira means alert firmness. We have to be alert. We cannot doze off. There are many techniques to develop sthira and sukha.

Question: Will you please review the concept of rāga?

Response: We need certain things in life. We are required to do certain things in life, otherwise, what is the purpose of being born? Unfortunately, all of us go one step further. We crave things and this craving has no relationship to our true needs or our aspirations in life. For example, I have a very good wrist watch in Madras. Yet the other day I was in one of your supermarkets and I saw a beautiful watch. What happens? Despite the fact that I already have a good watch, I want this one. I buy it. Again, on a trip to Switzerland I see a beautiful watch and a friend says he will buy it for me. Why not? Both of these examples are moments of rāga. While there is no harm in having something if we need it, we are always seeking things that have no relationship to need or purpose in life. This seeking can become a habit. We are besieged with gimmicks and advertisements to attract us. Why do we have such advertisements? To encourage rāga. To possess many gadgets doesn't mean we have a better life. Other things are more important. This is why rāga is undesirable. If we need things it is right to have them, but it is wrong to have them just because they are available.

Let us discuss the whole concept of yoga practice starting with a more detailed explanation of avidyā. We have said everything is changing, including avidyā. Avidyā is changing whether it shows itself as asmitā, rāga, dveṣa, or abhiniveśa. The manifestation of avidyā is not always the same. For example, sometimes it will show itself as fear, and sometimes there might be no fear but some other aspect. This could be desire, possessiveness, dislike, etc. The four aspects of avidyā are not always in balance. While all are usually present some will be prominent and others recessive. If we temporarily feel humble, it does not mean that we have conquered ego. We never know when a particular form of avidyā might arise. It is like planting seeds. The moment they get water, fertilizer, and air, they sprout. These differences express themselves at different times and they follow their own fashion. In some situations ego might dominate, in others, desire. We should never relax when we appear to have no avidyā. If these four aspects of avidyā are not always on the surface, we must be aware that their potency and depth change. Sometimes avidyā in its various expressions is very feeble, sometimes it is overpowering. Since there are many levels of avidyā, we must be very careful not to slacken our efforts, or our alertness and attention to action. If for a number of years there is a high level of clarity, there is good movement towards higher discovery. But suddenly, avidyā might come upon us like an earthquake. Therefore, we emphasize that this movement towards understanding, this practice, which we call yoga, must go on and on until avidyā is reduced to a minimum. A few days of āsana practice and self-inquiry might help for a short period of time, but it will never help forever. Practice is cumulative and gradual. We have to strive constantly towards perfection in these things because the word "better" controls our actions. We can be better than yesterday, but we can be worse tomorrow. So we must move continually until the seed that is called avidyā is burnt and cannot flower. As long as the germ is there, we never know whether or not it will sprout. The whole movement of yoga is to permanently destroy this seed called avidyā.

Avidyā relates to action. Whether this action is

good or bad, there is no question of not acting in life. Even our failure to act has results. This is very important because, depending upon the power or potency of avidyā, our actions will have positive or negative effects. The results of our actions show whether they were timely or proper. Action is understood to be of two types. One type is action that reduces avidyā and brings understanding from the puruṣa, and therefore, true understanding. The other type is action that increases avidyā. We can either increase avidyā by nurturing it or we can reduce it by starvation. Thus our actions can serve to encourage or discourage avidyā. Everything we do in yoga, whether it is āsana, prāṇāyāma, dhyāna, steady observation or inquiry, aims at reducing avidyā.

Any action we take might show its result immediately or in the course of time. An action can have an immediate good or bad result. An action can also leave a "residue" which might affect later actions. Therefore, it is a continuous process; one action influencing the other ad infinitum. This is why we must be very careful during the whole process of action. One way we could prevent negative actions, actions we might regret, is called dhyāna. In this context the word dhyāna means to reflect. This reflection may occur when we plan a course of action, and then imagine its exact opposite. We can then see what the result of this reverse action would be. Whether it is an action involving the practice of āsana or self study or a fundamental decision in life; even when we are very sure of our planned action, it is at this moment that we must reflect. We must imagine the extreme opposite course of action and its ramifications. Then we come back to our original plan to see how certain we are. This dhyāna is a type of quiet meditation through which we can avoid certain regrettable action. It affords us the occasion to examine our actions from a distance.

This reinforces another important aspect in yoga, independence. Yoga makes us svatantra. Sva means "self." Tantra means "technique." We use our own system, our own methods. We all like to be independent, yet, many of us are dependent on others, psychologists, gurus, teachers, drugs, etc. While consultation and guidance is a help, there is no doubt that finally we are the best judge of our own actions. No one is more interested in me than I, myself. This is the concept of dhyāna, the examination of the opposite view as a means of avoiding regrettable actions.

Question: Dhyāna, as reflection, involves the idea that yoga works towards independence. This reflection is some sort of imaginative effort to understand what might happen should we act in an opposite manner. Doesn't the result of my imaginative effort come from what I have gathered from others, observing their actions and the subsequent repercussions? In that way doesn't this work against the idea of yoga working independently? Why shouldn't I act and see what happens to me?

Response: When we are about to act and we take time to reflect, who is doing this reflection--ourselves. It is based upon our memory. What is memory--what we have seen, heard, or in any way experienced. But remember, our memory is not exactly what we have experienced but how we have interpreted it. Therefore, there is a part of ourselves in this process. What is very important in this concept of dhyāna is, at the moment we are about to act, we reflect. That reflection gives us additional time. With this time, we can improve the quality of our action. Not only can we reflect upon an opposite image, we can use another technique, pratipakṣa, in order to see things clearly. Pratipakṣa is removing ourselves from the situation by doing something completely different. Take the problem of my coming to Hamilton, New York. It was a big decision. Considering my work, my friends, my studies, it seemed foolish to leave Madras to work in Hamilton. On the other hand, it seemed so important to give these lectures that I had almost made a decision to go. Would this decision be a good one? At such a moment and after much thought it is better not to discuss Hamilton versus Madras. I went to a concert instead. Here there was no conflict. In this environment I made a decision to go to Hamilton. How did this process work? Even though I am at a concert or going for a ride, or whatever, subconsciously my mind is working without external pressure. At the concert I gain a distance. Subconsciously my mind is working, so I have time. However short it is, I am given time to have one more look at this whole decision I have to make. Perhaps I will then make a better decision. The time we get in dhyāna is extremely important in that we can reflect and through this reflection gain quality of action.

Question: Is it fair to say that in considering the alternatives, we allow the quality of our action to improve?

Response: Naturally, and we do this by any means, including dhyāna and pratipakṣa.

Question: How can we tell when our action is resulting from the puruṣa or from avidyā?

Response: When we feel like acting very quickly, when we feel we must do this or that, our actions result from avidyā. When we feel pressure to act, there is always avidyā. Seeing by the puruṣa involves quietness with alert understanding. When we have seen something clearly it is unhurried. When there is clarity, there is no pressure to act.

In the context of what we have been discussing I would like now to introduce the concept called duḥkha. Duḥkha is a disturbance of the mind. While sometimes the words sorrow, misery, and disease are used to define duḥkha, it is best identified as a feeling of restriction. Somehow something deeply disturbs us and we feel restricted. This restriction is duḥkha. When we feel a lot of space, have a sense of comfort and openness, that is the opposite, sukha. At different moments in everybody's life there is duḥkha. This concept is not only important to yoga but is also important in the other major philosophical systems of India. We all aim to remove duḥkha. That is what the Buddha taught. That is what Vedānta calls for. That is what yoga is trying to do. Duḥkha is the state of mind where we feel restricted from acting and seeing. While we may not show our emotions with rolling tears, somehow, deep within us, we feel disturbed. What is the relationship between *duḥkha* and *avidyā*? Any action resulting from *avidyā* always leads us to one or another form of *duḥkha*. Very often we might not see our *avidyā* expressed as ego, desire, hatred, or fear, but we recognize *duḥkha*. *Duḥkha* can express itself in different forms. We never know how it might express itself. Sometimes we feel choked, sometimes it is mental. No matter what form it takes, *duḥkha* is present at one moment or another when our actions result from *avidyā*. An action done with clarity from the *puruṣa* cannot have *duḥkha*. There are actions that somehow never have a negative aspect, and there are other actions which we thought were good but we came to regret.

Duḥkha comes about in a vicious circle. When we see something that we want and are able to get it, there is no *duḥkha*. If we are unable to get it, this is the beginning of *duḥkha*. Very often people have this type of *duḥkha* even when they are trying to improve their lives. They become so thirsty for understanding that they are unable to get understanding as quickly as they desire. In our great verses in Sanskrit, Tamil, as well as in other Indian literature, we have many stories about people striving to improve themselves. They are in such a hurry without results that they develop *duḥkha*. This form of *duḥkha* in which we see something we want but are unable to have is called *pariṇāma-duḥkha*. *Pariṇāma-duḥkha* might also be when we feel out of place in a new situation. For example, I am not used to American customs and I am unable to understand the people. I feel uneasy. Another example: I see a good camera in the shop. I want to buy it. I don't have the money with me. How I wish someone could lend me the money. There is also *tāpa duḥkha*. It is best explained through an example. I am used to Indian dishes as they are cooked in Madras. Though the same dishes can be prepared by wonderful cooks here, they are not as good as those prepared by my mother. So I am sitting here thinking, ah . . ., how I wish I had some of her *iddli* and only her *iddli*. Failing this, I cannot be satisfied. *Tāpa* is like thirst. Another form of *duḥkha* is *saṃskāra-duḥkha*. We are used to certain things and we can't do without them. We are conditioned to certain habits and when these habits are disturbed, we feel uneasy. This form of duḥkha comes from our own actions. Our actions have put us into grooves that make us happy and comfortable. When we can't continue in them, we are disturbed. Some of our grooves we know are not right, yet the process of coming out of these grooves is also duḥkha. That is why it is sometimes difficult to stop a particular action we recognize as bad. The separation from a habitual movement is very painful. It disturbs us. We try to identify these disturbances of the mind and to remove them.

There is one final aspect of duḥkha which is difficult to explain. The mind has three qualities or guṇas. They are tamas, rajas, and sattva. Tamas is heaviness. We feel dull. We want to do something but we put it off. For example, if it is time for me to give this lecture and at that moment I have heaviness, this will produce conflict and duḥkha. This lethargic quality of the mind is tamas. It is time to go to bed and rest, yet the mind says let us go out, let us go to a cinema, we must go to the cinema, how can we not go to the cinema? This quality of the mind wants to move, wants to dance. It is called rajas and also produces duḥkha. The third quality of the mind is really the absence of these two. There is no heaviness, no rush, there is only clarity. The mind is truly clear. This is called sattva and obviously it does not produce duḥkha. Thus of the three qualities or guṇas inherent to the mind, two are negative and one is positive. They have their own cycles of emphasis. At one time tamas may be strongest, at another time rajas or sattva.

In the combined effect of our habits and the quality of our minds there is always one type of disturbance or another. We try to reduce these through the practice of yoga.

Question: Is it sometimes better to try to have duḥkha?

Response: How? Can you elucidate?

Reply: Can we strive for duḥkha in order that we

might perceive something which, without this pain, we would not recognize or be motivated to change?

Response: Can you give an example?

Reply: For example, people who have duḥkha as a result of striving for perfection and are unable to achieve it.

Response: Yes, we must recognize duḥkha to remove it. But in my example the people are not bringing the duḥkha on themselves. They have duḥkha because they are unable to understand the truth despite their yoga practice. This is because they are in such a hurry they have duḥkha. In yoga one of the first levels of prajñā, wisdom, is the awareness and understanding that we are disturbed. It is the first truth we need to understand because very often duḥkha goes unrecognized. The first clarity in life is to see that we have duḥkha and then to do something about it. Therefore, we should not encourage duḥkha, we should discover that which is already there.

Duḥkha does not mean pain. It is a quality of mind where we feel more or less suffocated. It is unlike physical pain. We can cut our finger and this does not bother us mentally because we know we will be all right. There might be no physical pain and still be great duḥkha. Don't take the word duḥkha literally to mean pain. Another example--ten days ago I fell and hurt my knee. It was quite painful and I could barely bend my leg. It did not bother me because I knew I would be all right. Yet there are often small things buried within us that constantly bother us. It can be something very abstract or very subjective; but it is always in the "back of our head." That is duḥkha. It is a disturbance deep within us. If we have a craving for something, where is the pain? Can we show it in the body? Sometimes painful symptoms will appear. For example, sometimes a person who habitually smokes will develop a cough if he can't smoke. This physical pain is insignificant compared to duḥkha which is of the mind. While duḥkha might have physical results, it is primarily mental. Further we don't need to bring it out because it will show itself naturally. It is indeed rare to find someone who is never disturbed.

Question: If duḥkha is always present and wisdom is to realize this, then in a way, isn't that bringing it out?

Response: Yes. When we recognize duḥkha and that it is important to do something about it, we are able to find a way to be rid of it. This is why recognition of duḥkha is the first step towards clarity.

Question: In the face of a reality in which everything is in flux, everything is fleeting, a world which is constantly changing, we desire something which is there and always will be there. Is it this reality of the fleetingness of things which gives rise to our duḥkha?

Response: If we thought something was not changing and we established our lives on that basis and then gradually recognized that things were changing, we might have duḥkha. The opposite might also be the case. If we felt that everything was constantly changing, and therefore, we did nothing to establish anything in our lives, this might produce duḥkha. Yoga suggests that we have differing emphasis and relationships to all things. We must be flexible. Things are changing and therefore it is better to be flexible. Nothing is constant, but all things are reality. When we say that things are changing, it does not mean that this table will appear different tomorrow. Appearances change, not because of changing physical forms, but because of the change in our relationship to them. There is a human state called kaivalya. That is, a person is free. When a person is free, it means that things outside of himself are not as disturbing as they were in the past. Suppose I have a radio that I like very much. One day my son breaks it. I am shocked and angry with him even though he didn't deliberately do it. Yet, I shouldn't have gotten angry--the radio was broken. While I would not encourage my son to break things, I must be flexible. A little flexibility always reduces duḥkha.

Question: Can this be practiced? You said that you

have to begin by recognizing where we are. Is that connected with a recognition of duḥkha?

Response: Yes. Suppose we have a particular conception or notion about āsanas, why we should do āsanas, where we should begin, how long we should practice, etc. Then we make an investigation of how our breathing is, how our body is and through this we see that our starting point is different from our original concept. We must then change our plans and in so doing, we will reduce duḥkha.

There are so many outstanding books on āsanas, some containing very difficult postures. We might look at one of these books and think that we must do all the listed postures. When we don't know the condition of our hips, backs, legs, etc., when we don't know our starting point and we try to do these postures, we might end up with problems. In other books we are told how to do prāṇāyāma. They say the best prāṇāyāma is breathing in through one nostril and breathing out through the other. We are told to use a ratio of one for inhalation, four for holding the breath, two for exhalation, and one for holding the breath. For example, inhale six counts, hold the breath twenty-four counts, exhale twelve counts, hold the breath six counts. If we can inhale sixteen counts, hold the breath sixty-four counts, exhale thirty-two counts, and hold the breath sixteen counts, we will be as free as a bird. Unfortunately, many try this and not only end up with a chest pain, they might feel strange. The differing interpretations of yoga found in so many recent books, and the great exposure we have to so many ideas, makes it even more important for us to know how to investigate ourselves in everything we do. I have one master and I have been with him for sixteen years. He knows me very well. Because of this relationship, whatever he tells me, I know I can accept. For most people, it is not like that. This is why we must investigate where we are--whether it is for āsana, breathing or the study of the whole concept of yoga. Otherwise, there will be more duḥkha. Less duḥkha means something disturbs us less, more duḥkha means something disturbs us more.

Question: What causes duḥkha?

Response: The cause of duḥkha is avidyā.

For those of you who want to do some related reading on yoga, the basis for these lectures will be the second chapter of Patañjali's Yoga Sūtra.

IV

Practice

PRACTICE PLANNING

In the second lecture, the first on practice, I discussed the meaning of āsana, how breathing is important to postures, how to coordinate breathing with movement, what is proper breathing and the reason for this technique. The importance of planning a practice was also introduced. Are there any questions?

Question: If we started doing yoga on our own, doing all the postures daily without paying attention either to breathing or to how we are doing the postures, is that worthless?

Response: I'm sure it would help to make us supple, but there can be dangers. There are some people who seem able to do all the āsanas but know nothing about their bodies and limitations. Often these people end up needing help to overcome injuries caused by their unguided enthusiasm. For example, a person might do a deep bending backward posture and, not knowing proper preparation and compensation, end up with a slipped disc. Then there is another problem. I had one student who could do all the āsanas and was shocked to discover that she was unable to stay in mahā mudrā for eight breaths! She was so flexible that she took her body for granted. Mahā mudrā requires more than suppleness of the body. We must be able to stay and breathe in this posture. (See Figure 15.)

There is another problem. By training in calisthenics or gymnastics, a person can become so supple that he can do almost anything. What is it that makes yoga āsanas different from this? Will someone who knows nothing about yoga recognize the difference between it and gymnastics or calisthenics merely by looking at a book on yoga āsanas? I doubt it unless the way we organize the course, breathing, the way we pay attention to breathing and movement in the

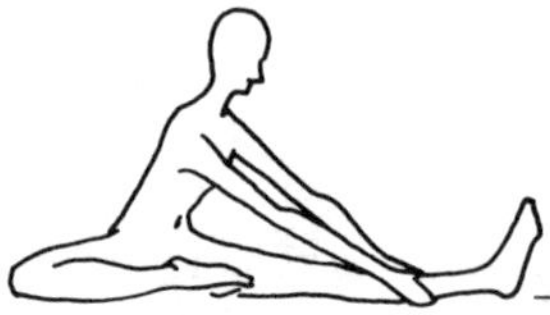

mahā mudrā

Fig. 15

posture will itself make the difference. Throughout any activity in yoga, there must be attention to what we are doing. Yoga, unlike dance or mime, is not an expression of form for others to watch. We are doing it for ourselves. We are the observers and we are the observed. What we observe is posture. We can see this in our group classes. Each person becomes so involved in his or her own breath and flexibility that he or she will not be aware of outsiders. In yoga āsanas we observe what we are doing, not the outside, and no one outside observes for us. If this aspect is missing, if there is no self attention, it is difficult to call it yoga. We will go into this as we go into planning.

It is important that yoga practice be planned in a sensible, organized way. When we practice āsanas, as with anything in life, we have a starting point. Our condition before beginning the practice, which we discover through some investigation, is this starting point. We then ascend gradually; that is, we prepare the body by warming up, getting proper breathing started, etc. After we slowly ascend to the "crown" or apex of our day's practice, we slowly descend. This is the concept of yoga practice,

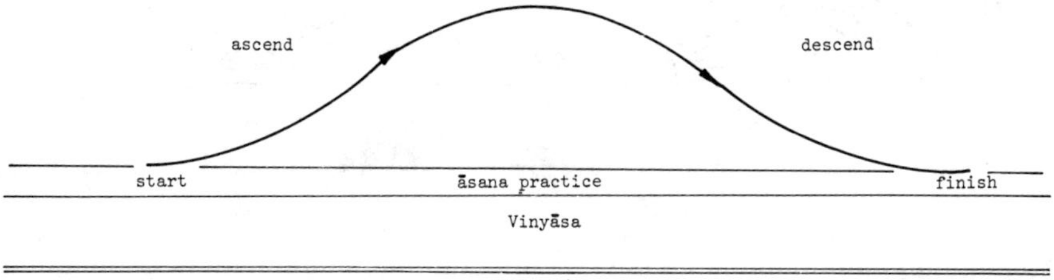

Fig. 16

whether it is āsanas, prāṇāyāma, or any other aspect. We start where we are, gradually ascend and then descend. Suppose we do the headstand and then stop our practice abruptly. We may feel dizzy, we may get stiff necks. Not only must we ascend to a particular point, we must come back to a point from which we can function in the world. This applies to the practice of a single āsana as well as the progress of an entire sequence spanning a year. The point to be emphasized is that we should proceed very gradually. If in cold weather we cannot easily do paścimatānāsana (sitting, bending forward), we should not try to force our legs and push our heads down to attain the posture. There is no need, nor will there be any profit. Wait. Little by little the body will give in. We must always go by progressions in yoga. Each day's practice must have a gradual ascent and descent. There is one more point. The way we plan a course will also depend, in addition to the starting point, upon our activities following the course. A course of āsanas designed to prepare the body to play ten-

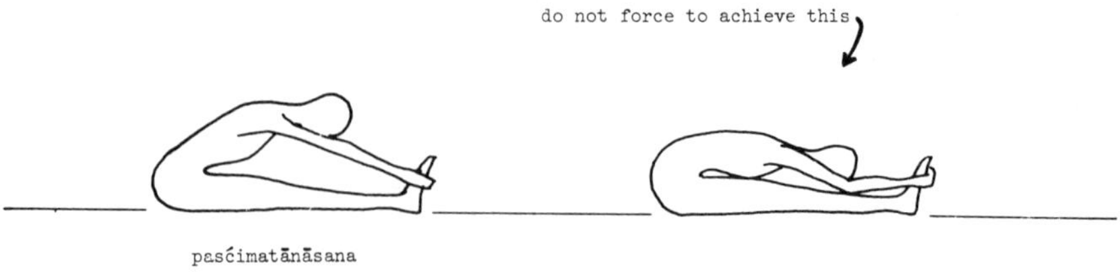

Fig. 17

nis will be different from a course designed to help us relax without being drowsy in the office.

Question: Are you saying that the starting point is different every day? If one day I have a stuffy nose or a bad knee or anything else, should I work with these problems?

Response: Yes. It may be difficult in the beginning. The more we expose ourselves to practice, the more we will understand how we can observe ourselves and how to discover our starting point. The starting point is variable. I have hurt my knee. I can't sit cross-legged in the morning; therefore, I must do postures that will work toward limbering up my injured knee. It is very important to investigate our condition before we practice. For example, if we stand and bend forward, we will know if our legs and backs are stiff. Some things are very obvious if we start watching. Once we observe and know our starting point, we can plan our practice. With a little intelligence,

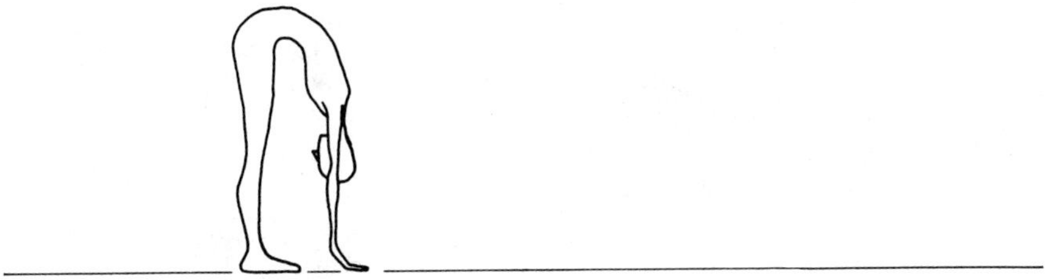

Fig. 18

we will always find a way. Suppose tomorrow we want to do upaviṣṭha koṇāsana (sitting with legs spread, bending forward). In order to do this we have to find out what is involved in this posture. There are many areas that need preparation: we have to bend the trunk, loosen the hips, stretch between and under the legs, stretch the back, contract the stomach and be able to breathe in this bent position. If we understand these things, we create certain steps which will help us to be really comfortable in this posture. Then we have reached our goal.

In Sanskrit, this concept of intelligently conceived steps in order to reach a desired point is called vinyāsa. If we want to do a particular posture, we need to find out what is involved in the posture, then prepare the body and breath so that the posture can be done without strain. In planning a sequence of āsanas there must be preparation. Suppose we want to do padmāsana (lotus posture, sitting, knees bent with feet resting on opposite thighs). We know we can't use the same steps as in upaviṣṭha koṇāsana. We

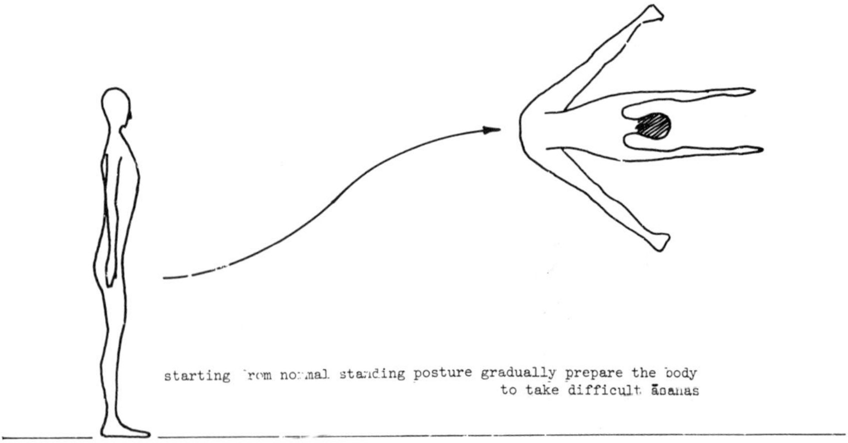
starting from normal standing posture gradually prepare the body to take difficult āsanas

concept of vinyāsa

Fig. 19

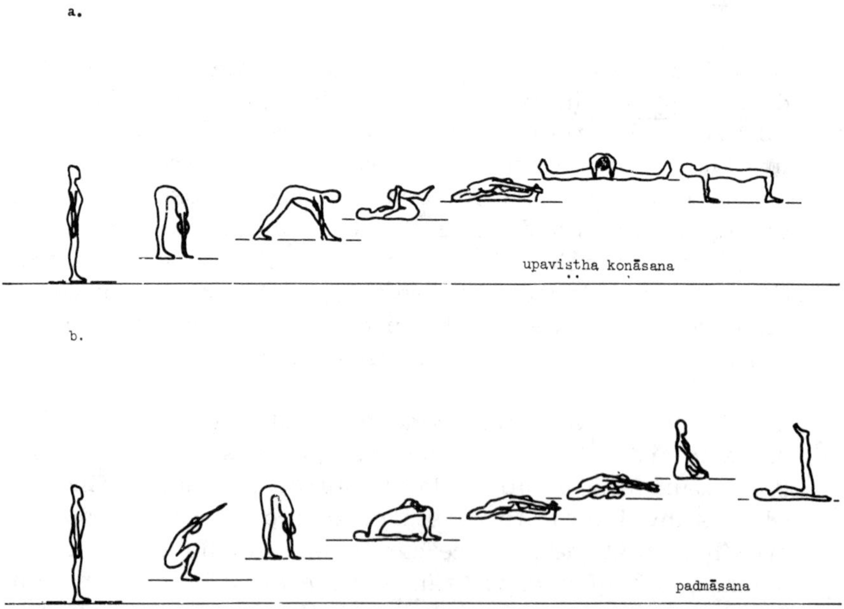
a.
upaviṣṭha koṇāsana
b.
padmāsana

Vinyāsa depends on the āsana we aim for.

Fig. 20a,b

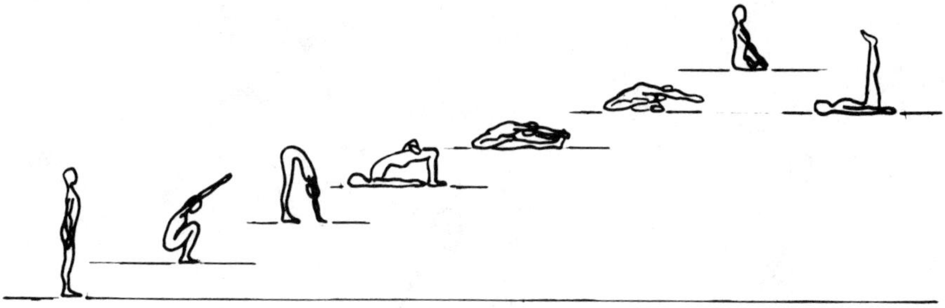

Vinyāsa depends on the āsana we aim for.

Fig. 20b

don't have to stretch the legs in a lotus position, but we do have to twist the hips and the knees and limber up our ankles. We can do this preparation with utkaṭāsana (squat posture). Then uttānāsana (standing, bending forward). Then a knee variation in the posture dvipāda pīṭham (desk pose). Then possibly some posture like ardha padma paścimatānāsana (sitting in half-lotus, bending forward) for twisting the knee and hip towards padmāsana. With this preparation, perhaps we can get into the lotus position. If we can't, we will wait until tomorrow or however long it takes. Postures must not inflict torture. We must take steps that will make up happy, sukha, to be in a posture. For this, intelligent steps are required.

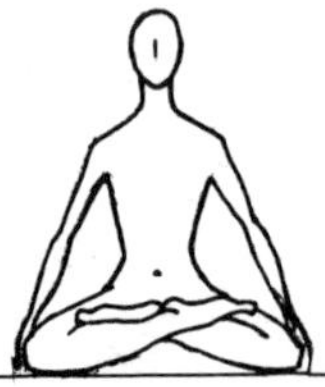

padmāsana

Fig. 21

There is another example, the well-known śīrṣāsana (headstand). We begin on our feet, and we have to move to a point where we are on our heads. This means the neck will be taking a lot of weight. The effects of gravity must be considered. We must gradually prepare ourselves so that we are at ease in the headstand. How do we achieve this? We must begin with some warm-up postures, then something for the neck, and perhaps something inverted, so that we get used to this position. While preparation is important, another important point to explain is the descent from a posture or its compensation. Compensation is to counter the negative effects of a posture. I have an interesting story about compensation. I have two brothers. When we were children we had very tall coconut trees in our yard. My older brother said he knew how to climb tall

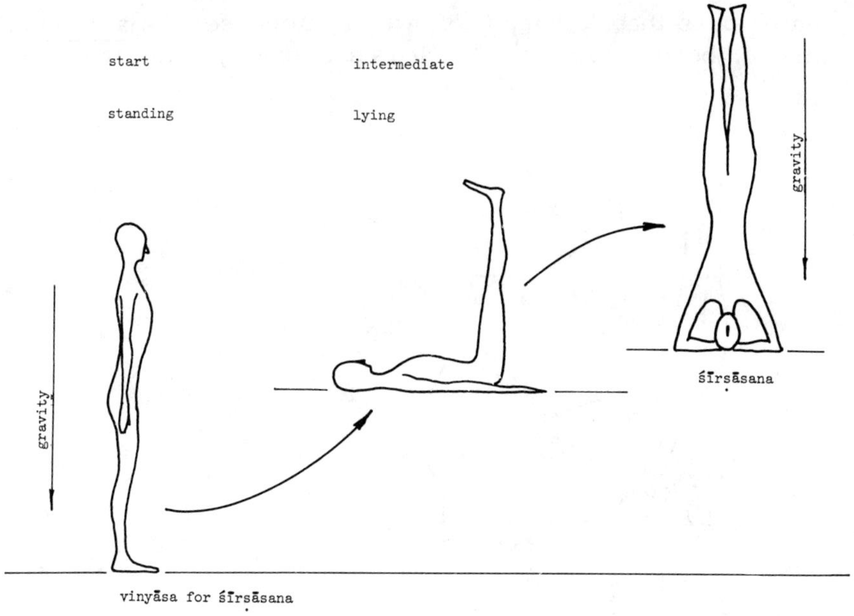

Fig. 22

trees, so my other brother and I challenged him to do it. I distinctly remember taunting him to "go up, go up, go up." He climbed the tree but he did not know how to come down. There was no one to help him so he remained there for quite some time. This is what we mean by compensation. It is not enough to climb the tree, we must know how to come down. When we do a headstand, we should be able to come back to a normal position without problems. We call such compensation a counterpose. In my brother's case, the positive effect was that he could climb the tree. The negative effect was that he could not come down. In a similar way, we must keep the positive effect of a posture and eliminate the negative effect. When we teach the headstand, we first teach preparation, then we teach the counterpose sarvāṅgāsana (shoulder stand) which in itself is a major pose that demands its own counterpose bhujaṅgāsana (prone, bending backward). It is all very systematic. Plan-

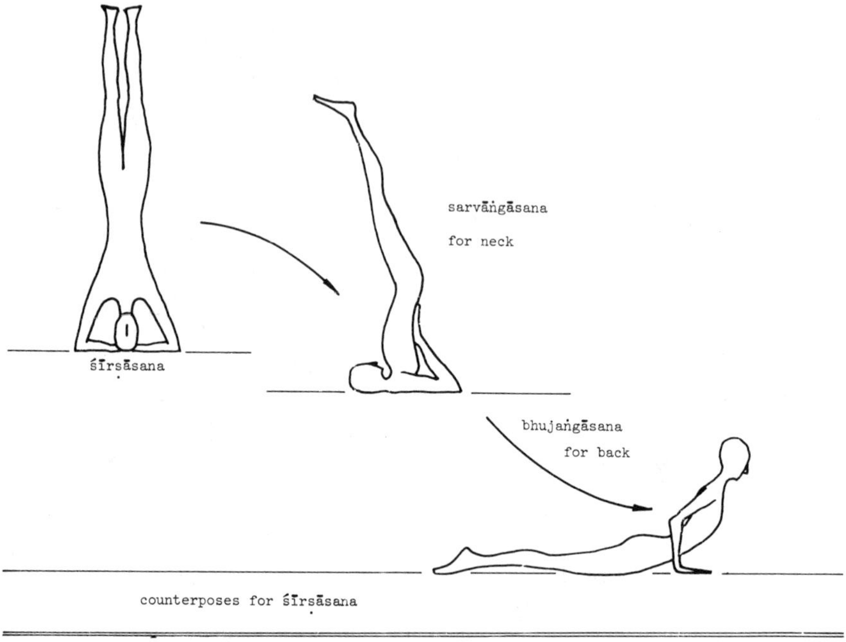

Fig. 23

ning means to go gradually, to prepare, and then to compensate. Preparation and compensation are unnecessary when postures compensate each other. We can plan our practice so that sometimes this mutual compensation, so important to our work, is present.

Certain principles govern our preparation. We should begin with postures that bend the body in a natural way. As an example, it is not good to begin by bending backward, twisting, or doing headstands. We should always start with the simplest things; raising the arms, bending the body forward, raising one leg while lying down, etc. Start with the easiest and little by little we can introduce the more difficult.

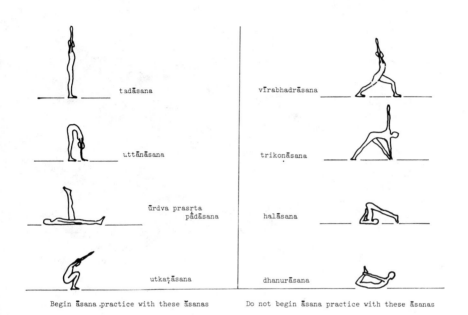

Fig. 24

When we do a posture, we must counter it immediately. This we call compensation. The moment we feel a strain in any area of our body, we must try to compensate through some counterpose. There could be different counterposes for the same posture, depending upon where the strain is felt. For example:

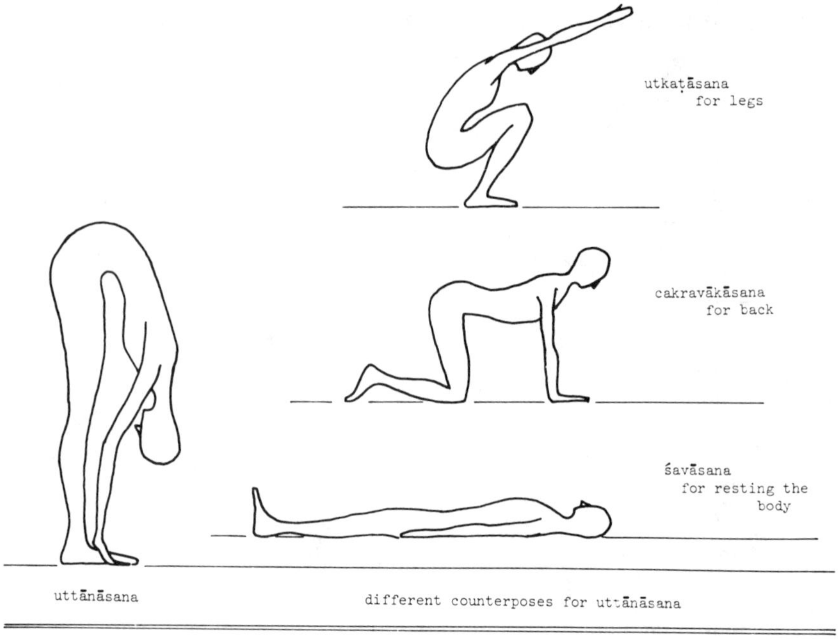

Fig. 25

The counterpose for a given strain is generally the easiest pose opposite to the direction of the strain. When we do a deep bending forward posture, the counterpose that compensates is a gentle bending backward posture. When we do a deep bending backward posture, the counterpose is a gentle bending forward posture. When we do a twisting posture, the counterpose is a simple bending forward posture. The reason we do this is to return the body to a normal condition. In special postures like the headstand, we must find out just where the strain is felt and compensate accordingly. In the example of the headstand some of us need to compensate for pain in the lower back if we have a hollow back. Others need to compensate for the strain on the neck. The counterpose for a given posture is not always the same. The counterpose is decided by the effect

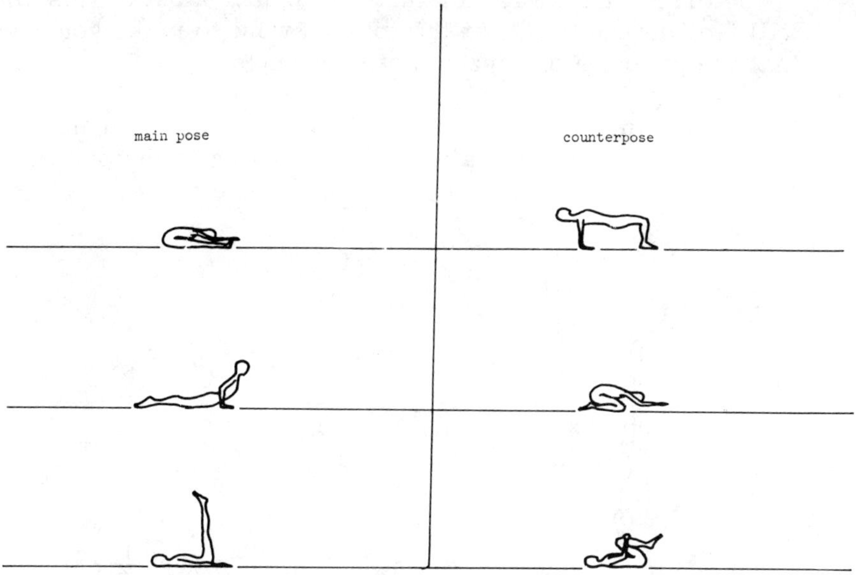

Examples for counterpose

Fig. 26

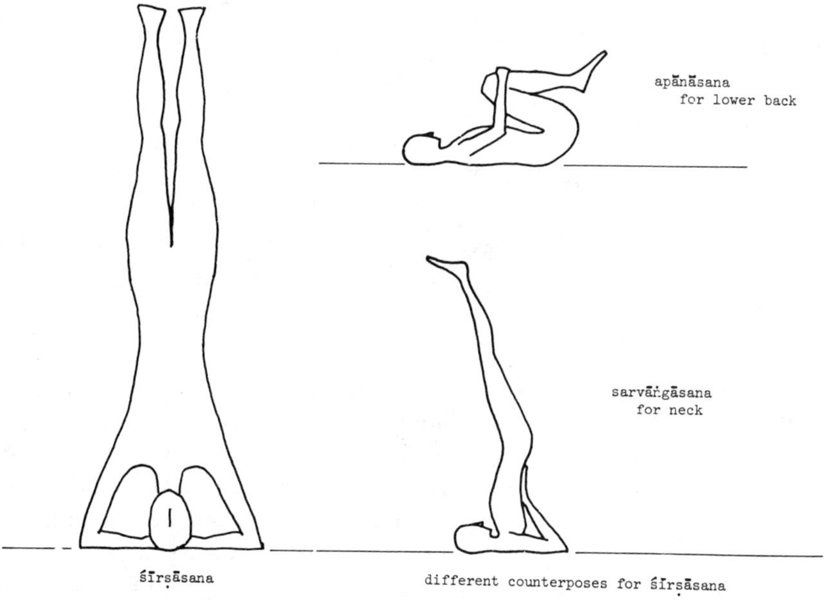

Fig. 27

of the original pose rather than its form. Most of this you will feel in practice. At this point I want to make you aware that the practice of yoga is not haphazard.

Postures can be done in two ways, either dynamically through repetition or statically, by staying in the posture for some time. For example, paścimatānāsana:

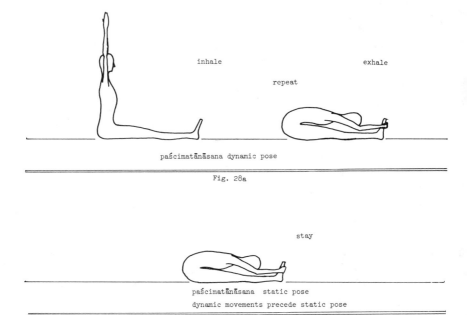

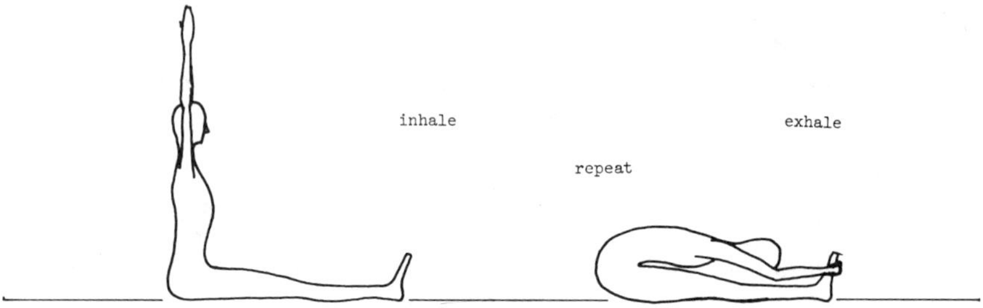

paścimatānāsana dynamic pose

Fig. 28a

paścimatānāsana static pose

dynamic movements precede static pose

Fig. 28b

It is always better to do a posture dynamically before we try to stay. This applies either to a single practice or a sequence of sessions. Dynamic movement always precedes static posture, thereby allowing the body to get used to the position, and compensate. These are some of the principles of a planned practice: start exactly where we are; prepare the body so that all the joints are limber; before doing a posture, make sure we know a counterpose; always do a counterpose after the main pose; the counterpose must always be easier than the main pose; do the pose dynamically before staying.

Rest is also important to our planning. Obviously we must rest if we become breathless or unable to control our breath. Even if our breath is under control and some part of our body becomes tired or sore, we must rest. So above all, when we need rest, we rest. If we plan to do a posture twelve times and we feel tired after six times, we must stop. Also, rest is used for transition. By transition we mean from one type of posture to another. For example, we rest between dhanurāsana (prone, holding ankles-bow posture), a deep bending backward posture and paścimatānāsana. We might not feel

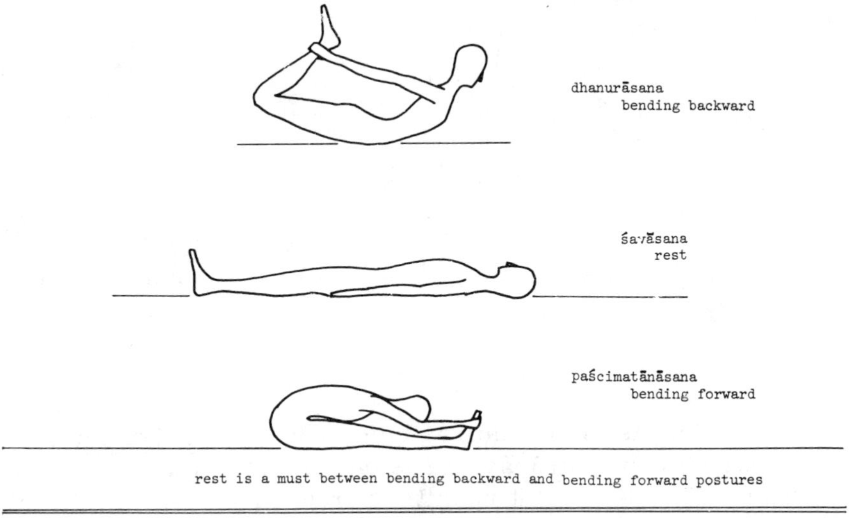

Fig. 29

the need, but we must rest. During rest periods we have a chance to feel the muscular effects of the posture, the muscles recoiling. In this case, if we don't rest, we might unknowingly strain our backs while doing the bending forward posture. To avoid this problem, we rest and while resting examine the reaction of our muscles.

Some people feel comfortable while in a headstand

but note a pressure on their chest when they lie down afterwards. In a headstand the whole weight of the abdomen is on the chest compressing the ribs. They do not notice this during the pose, but it appears when they lie down. The feeling of pressure on the chest is just the reaction of the ribs that should be relieved through a resting posture before doing the counterpose.

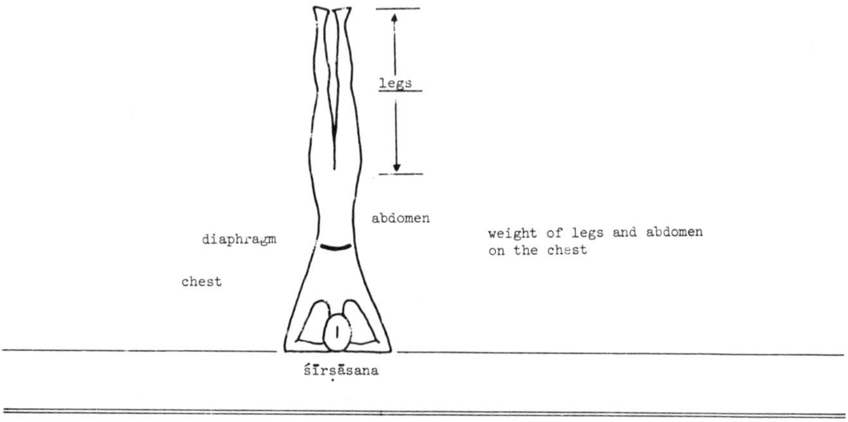

Fig. 30

Rest is also required before doing prāṇāyāma. The primary focus of prāṇāyāma is on the breath, while in āsanas breathing is dependent upon the particular posture. Since āsanas call for attention to the body, it is good to rest to prepare mentally for prāṇāyāma.

Question: How much rest should we have before prāṇāyāma?

Response: It depends on how many postures we have done. If we have done postures for about fifteen minutes, we will need two or three minutes rest. If we have practiced for an hour or more, we need at least five minutes rest. While doing āsanas there is always a tendency to rush; therefore, the more time spent doing āsanas, the more we rest.

Question: Is every movement from a main pose to a counterpose a transition?

Response: Yes, usually we have to rest. After a headstand, rest, then do a shoulderstand. If the counterpose is an easy one, we don't need to rest. For example:

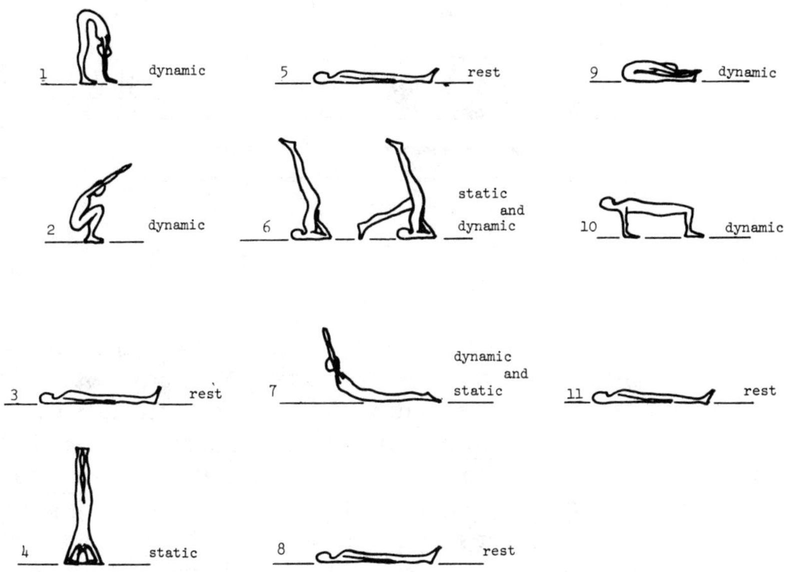

a sequence of āsanas indicating rest position

Fig. 31

Question: If we do two or three different standing postures in our warmups, do we need a counterpose between each one if they all involve a bending forward posture?

Response: Suppose I want to do the following:

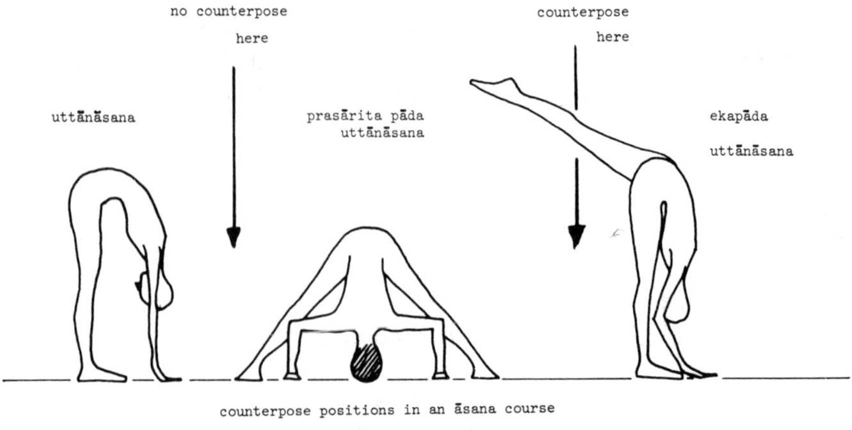

Fig. 32

All the āsanas involve leg stretching. Your question is, where should we do the counterpose? We may not need a counterpose after uttānāsana. We would definitely use one after prasārita pāda uttānāsana (standing with legs spread, bending forward). We should not wait until after eka pāda uttānāsana (standing, bending forward with one leg extended upwards). By then it might be too late. If after we have done the counterpose our legs still feel tired, we know that the counterpose was done too late or it was inadequate. It is better to err on the safe side and do a counterpose early when we are doing a series of bending forward postures.

I would like to tell you something about holding the breath in postures. There are four parts to breathing: inhalation, exhalation, and retention after inhalation and exhalation. In āsanas we should never hold the breath if it is going to reduce the length of the inhalation or exhalation. Sometimes holding the breath is useful. Holding the breath can be used to intensify the effect of a posture. Suppose we feel heavy in the abdominal region and we use uttānāsana to

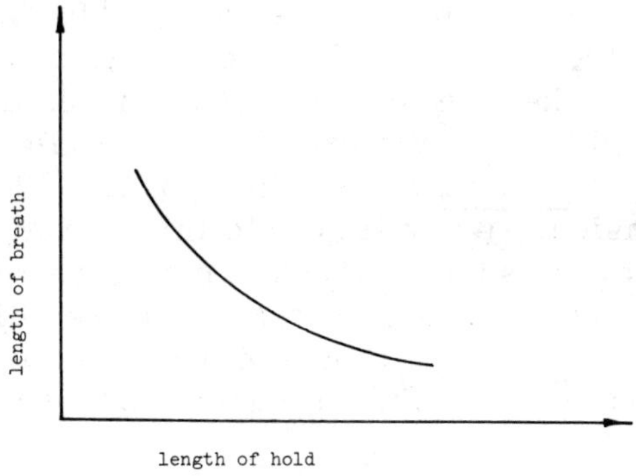

effect of retention on the length of breath

Fig. 33

help us feel lighter. We can do the posture in its simplest form, dynamically with slow breathing or we can go down on exhalation while pulling in the abdomen and remain down, holding the breath for five or six seconds. Such retention after exhalation increases the posture's effect on the abdomen. On the other hand, if we inhale and hold the breath the effect on the chest is increased. This is a basic principle of yoga. Long inhalations and holding of the breath after inhalation increases the effect on the chest. Long exhalation and holding of the breath after exhalation increases the effect on the abdomen. We use this principle of control of the breath to bring about different effects in our postures. In forward bending postures there is a tendency to hold the breath after exhalation. In backward bending postures, if we wish to increase their effect, we hold the breath after inhalation.

We can also use retention of the breath to increase the duration of inhalation and exhalation; that is, holding the breath after we inhale can be used to increase the length of inhalation, and holding the breath after we exhale can be used to increase the length of exhalation. In this, we must be careful. This is only a general principle, and under most circumstances the principle cannot be applied quite so simply. In Sanskrit this practice of making the exhalation longer and holding the breath after exhalation is called *laṅghana*. *Laṅghana* means "to fast." In this case we are "fasting" the lungs. Whenever there is a problem below the diaphragm, we do *laṅghana*. Likewise the concept of increasing the length of inhalation and holding the breath after inhalation is called *bṛmhaṇa*. *Bṛmhaṇa* means "to expand." We can literally feel this expansion. We will go into this in detail when we discuss *prāṇāyāma*. In short, *laṅghana* means to reduce; *bṛmhaṇa* to expand. *Laṅghana* means to remove the "dirt" in the abdomen; *bṛmhaṇa* means to have more effect on the chest and this is only a rule of thumb. In some cases we must make excep-

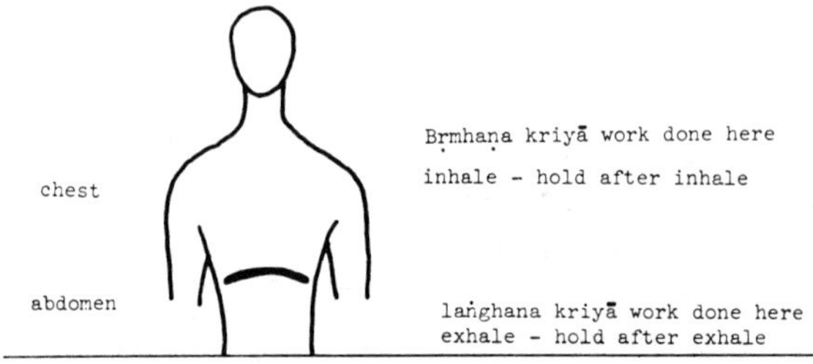

Bṛmhaṇa and Laṅghana kriyās

Fig. 34

tions for many reasons. Take the case of an asthmatic; it is foolish to ask him to hold the breath after inhalation--he cannot. In such a case, we only ask him to try to lengthen his exhalation. This basic principle must be used with understanding and not applied without careful consideration of particular circumstances.

Question: Should we try to hold our breath at all if it affects the steadiness of inhalation and exhalation?

Response: Holding the breath should never be done at the cost of inhalation and exhalation. In terms of the circulatory system, holding the breath should never be done if there is an abrupt increase in the rate of the heartbeat. Normally the heartbeat and respiration are balanced. If breathing is poor the pulse increases. So if the breath gets short, do not hold the breath. There are also psychological reasons for

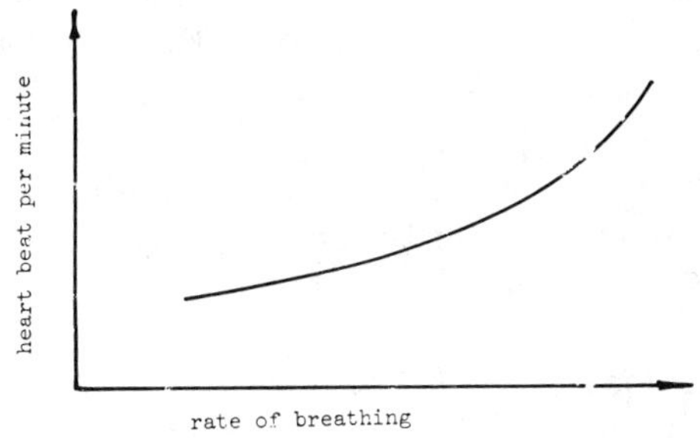

relationship between heart beat and breathing rate

Fig. 35

this rule. Some people are very nervous about their hearts, and a rapid increase in their pulse might cause anxiety. We already have enough anxiety. Holding the breath should never make us uneasy while controlling the quality of breathing.

Question: What time of day should we do our āsana practice?

Response: It depends upon the individual and the particular type of practice. We cannot say that practice times are fixed, such as morning or night. It is very important, however, to refrain from doing āsana practice after a meal. If we try to do a bending forward posture after eating, we will get cramps. If the stomach is full we cannot move the diaphragm well and our breathing cannot be completely controlled. Also, after a meal the whole body, circulation, etc., is concentrated upon digestion. When we do an exercise the circulation all over the body is equally involved. The gastric secretions used in digestion are formed through circulation; therefore, exercise will disturb digestion. We can practice about two or three hours after a meal. Some people wonder whether they can do āsanas during a long fasting session. This is bad because it will definitely disturb the liver. When we fast, the body is actually "eating itself." Mild breathing exercises may be all right or even useful but strong exercise might cause problems. For those people who have flexible schedules, it is best to practice in the morning before breakfast.

Question: If we do not have specific problems to consider in our practice, is there any way for us to know how many basic āsanas we should do each day, and which ones?

Response: If we know and enjoy doing the headstand, it can become the crown of our practice. Then the rest of our course can be built around the headstand, including all necessary preparation and counterposes. If we don't want to do a headstand, then the crown of our practice could be prāṇāyāma. We simply prepare the body for good breathing. This involves preparation for a seated posture. We don't waste time doing a lot of difficult backbends. We simply do āsanas so that our backs will be straight and our shoulders, necks, knees, and ankles will not be stiff. Then we examine our breathing. We use some arm movements or some trunk twisting to loosen the abdomen and ribs. Then we are ready for prāṇāyāma. What we do depends upon what we want to do. We don't need to do the headstand or any particular sequence every day. It is important to vary our practice to keep from getting bored. I will introduce many variations so you can experiment. This keeps up interest and there is always something new to discover.

Question: What sort of postures would be a good preparation for prāṇāyāma?

Response: To warm up, we might start with utkaṭāsana, holding the breath five seconds after inhalation and exhalation. Next we might do dvipāda pīṭham (supine, knees bent with feet on floor, trunk raised--desk pose) to prepare our backs, necks and to investigate our breathing. Then we might do cakravākāsana (knee, hand crawling position) (named after a mythological bird) for the chest and the back. With such preparation some of us can sit in sukhāsana (simple cross-legged posture), or failing this we can do prāṇāyāma sitting on a stool or straight chair. We won't lose anything by sitting on a chair though some have psychological inhibitions about this. This is the minimum preparation for doing prāṇāyāma. In any of

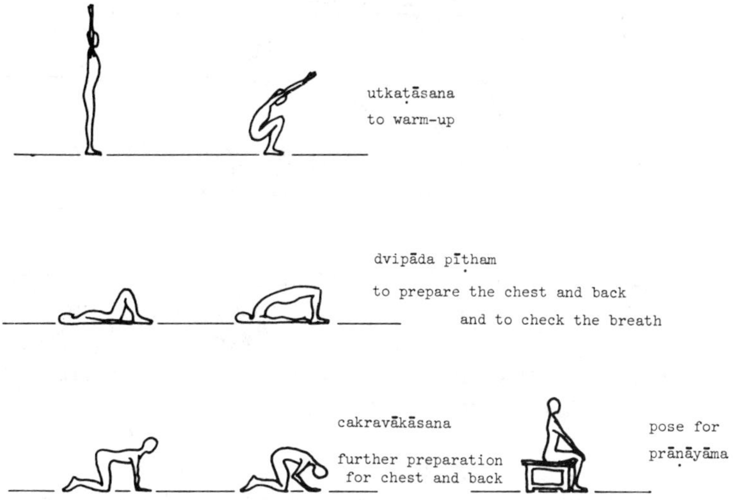

a typical course to prepare for prāṇāyāma

Fig. 36

these preparatory āsanas we can test our capacity to breathe as it might apply to a chosen prāṇāyāma. Take, for example, the ratio of inhale six seconds, hold the breath twenty-four seconds, exhale twelve seconds. Test this with the following āsana:

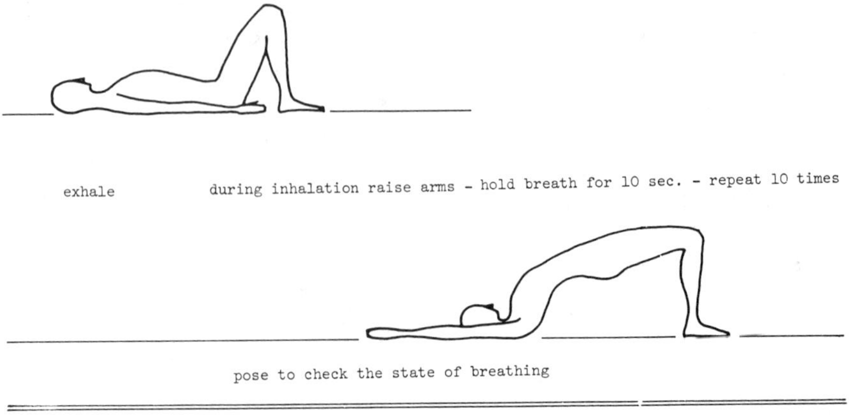
exhale
during inhalation raise arms - hold breath for 10 sec. - repeat 10 times
pose to check the state of breathing

Fig. 37

If we find that we cannot do this simple posture even ten times while holding the breath ten seconds after inhalation, we know we cannot do the more demanding ratio of 6:24:12. Again it must be stressed that the above program is minimal and that we can do much more if time permits.

Please don't have the idea that programs are fixed, that is, on Monday we do the headstand, on Tuesday we do the shoulderstand, etc. Programs are planned taking into consideration our free time, capabilities, and desires. We must always plan our practice as a unit, whether it is small or large. That means we start and finish in one session, at one particular time. If there is a chance that we are going to be disturbed or interrupted during our practice, it is better to plan a short course.

V

Theory

DUḤKHA AND THE CONCEPT OF SAṂSKĀRA

I have touched upon the notion of avidyā and its relationship to action. Positive actions are those that reduce avidyā and bring clarity; other actions are from avidyā. Some actions stemming from avidyā might not have negative results immediately, but in time, they will have detrimental repercussions. One action can influence another action until, in effect, we have little freedom to act. We simply continue in the same groove. In short, we don't really act, creatively act. I mentioned that action can result in a feeling called duḥkha; a feeling of restriction rather than freedom. I noted the various types of duḥkha. Pariṇāma-duḥkha results from not getting something we want. We see something, want it but can't have it. Tāpa-duḥkha results from a pleasant experience. We want to repeat it but it is now not possible. Saṃskāra-duḥkha results from becoming used to having something that we now can't have.

The Yoga Sūtra states that duḥkha is not always readily discerned by everyone, but only by those who seek clarity. There is a beautiful example given in Vyasa's commentary on the Yoga Sūtra. It says dust that blows on the skin is harmless, but if a tiny particle gets into the eye we suffer. In other words, a person who seeks clarity becomes sensitive like the eye. He feels or sees things before others do. It is a special kind of wisdom. This sensitivity acts like a yellow light before the red. It warns us that something disturbing is going to happen, so we are cautious. That is why there is always more apparent duḥkha for a viveki, one who is seeking clarity, than for someone who is not. This duḥkha results from greater sensitivity.

I also mentioned the three qualities (guṇas) of the mind. One is the quality of heaviness. Sometimes we don't feel like acting even when there are many things for us to do. The second quality is when the mind has to "dance." We can't keep ourselves quiet. The third quality of the mind is the absence of the first two. The combination of the heaviness and "dancing" of the mind results in different qualities of duḥkha.

Question: You referred to two of the three qualities of the mind which result in duḥkha. What about the third quality?

Response: When the mind doesn't have these qualities of heaviness or "dance," it is then characterized as having sattva-guṇa. Sattva means clarity. It is like a clean mirror. We aim to reduce the two adverse guṇas so that the mind becomes characterized by sattva. Yoga uses the Sanskrit word citta for mind and cit for the puruṣa. Citta means "that in us which thinks it is the thing that sees." Cit is "that which sees." On the periphery, there is something that thinks it sees. That is the citta. When the mind is free from heaviness or "dancing," it has the clarity of sattva-guṇa. An illustration would be helpful. The triangle is an outside object.

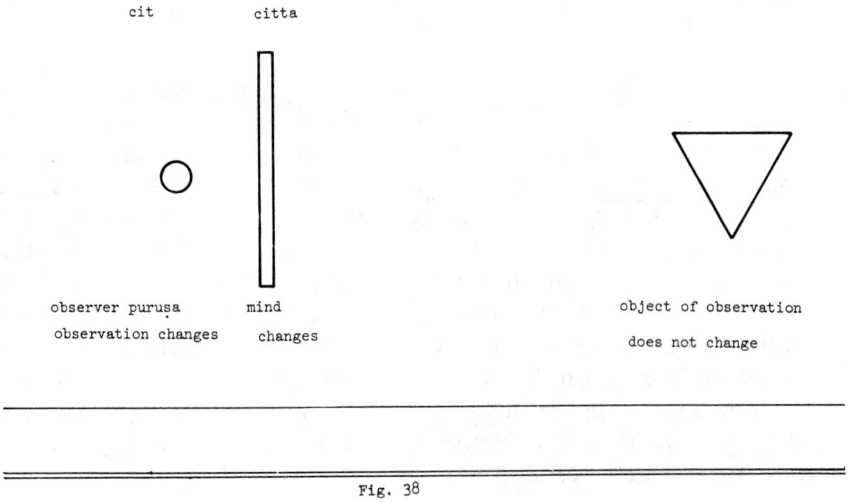

Fig. 38

The image of it falls on the mind so that the cit can see. If the mind is colored, the triangle appears colored to the cit.

If the mind is dusty, then there is no image at all. If the mind is clear, the cit sees the triangle as it is. If the mind has heaviness, it can't see; if the mind is unsteady or "dancing," the image is unclear; if the mind is neither heavy nor unsteady, it sees the image clearly.

To review, duḥkha can arise either from two of the three qualities of the mind or conditioning of the mind from avidyā. If the mind is clouded by avidyā, there will be duḥkha, a disturbance or a feeling of restriction.

Question: I don't understand how duḥkha becomes valuable for the person seeking clarity?

Response: It is a warning. It gives a person time to think. The more we seek clarity, the more sensitive we become, therefore, we observe more and see more, both positive and negative. On the other hand, the person who does not seek clarity does not know what brings happiness and what brings duḥkha.

Question: Is seeking clarity trying to see duḥkha?

Response: It is the first step. Yoga describes wisdom in seven steps. All of these steps are complicated except the first, which is an understanding of that which should be avoided. For example, we know that something is bothering us and that we must do something about it. We might not know what to do, but we recognize the problem. That is the first of the seven steps of wisdom, prajñā. Prajñā means wisdom, clarity, awareness. This condition of being bothered is much greater for a person who seeks understanding.

Question: Are dreams a form of duḥkha?

Response: To answer this question we must consider briefly the five faculties of the mind. (1) Pramāṇa is an activity of the mind that registers things accurately through the senses. (2) Viparyaya is an activity of the mind that registers things that are never accurately confirmed. (3) Vikalpa is imagination, that knowledge or understanding based purely on words and ideas with no substance or reality. (4) Nidrā is dreamless sleep. (5) Smṛti is memory, the activity of mind that retains the experience of an observation. These faculties of the mind work together. With the exception of nidrā, at any one moment there is likely to be a mixture of them. Any of these faculties or a combination of them is not necessarily a form of duḥkha but they have the possibility of affecting the amount of duḥkha. Dreams draw upon a combination of the faculties of the mind. Whether or not a dream brings duḥkha depends upon its effects. The effects of a dream might be good or bad, depending upon what we do with it or what it does to us. To help a disturbed mind, yoga recommends thinking about a pleasant dream; to remember and to investigate what aspects gave pleasure.

Question: In your diagram (Figure 38), how does the triangle or object interrelate with the citta (mind) and/or cit (puruṣa)?

Response: Think of the mind as a camera. The image of the object is projected on the mind through the lens of the senses, but the seeing is coming from the direction of cit (puruṣa). The puruṣa observes through the mind. If the

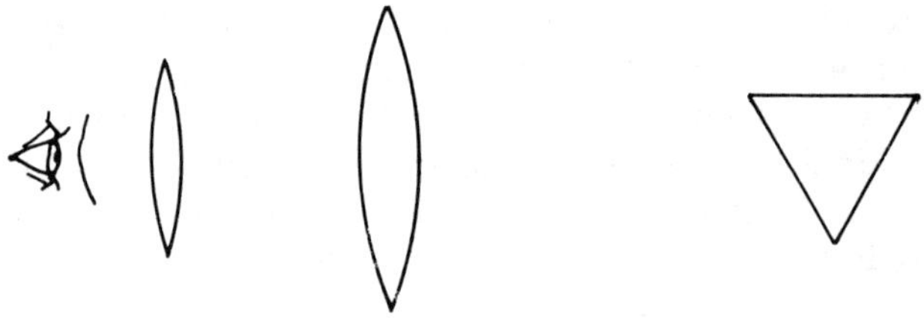

observation is similar to a view from a camera

Fig. 39

mind is colored the image is colored; if the mind is clear, the observation is perfect. Since the puruṣa can observe only through the mind, the quality of observation depends solely upon the state of mind. The mind is the instrument for the puruṣa to see. The puruṣa, in fact, provides the power for the mind to function. This is very important. The mind cannot see by itself. The energy and power to see is given to the mind only by the puruṣa. The impression that the puruṣa sees depends upon the quality of the mind. That is why in yoga we work with the mind. We can't do anything with the puruṣa. If we make the mind steadily clearer, the observations by the puruṣa get steadily clearer.

Question: If the energy for seeing comes from the puruṣa but the quality of seeing is determined by the state of mind, is it the mind that decides where to focus our attention?

Response: Very often the mind does make that decision. While it should not, it does, because it has been conditioned to do so. We called that saṃskāra, constant and automatic movement of the mind in a particular direction. This is why some of the practices we do in yoga are so important. In āsanas, for example, we do some exercises that are not conditioned by our usual mental activities and yet are not beyond our capabilities. We make a plan to do this practice and during its execution, perhaps, the mind is clear. When this happens, there is some clarity, and we might find that we have to change our plan. This sense of reorientation is communicated in the Sanskrit term parivṛtti. Suppose we are driving a car and there is a tree directly ahead. We anticipate hitting the tree and we steer the car in a slightly different direction. This seeing a bit ahead and redirection is what is meant by the concept of parivṛtti. Instead of the mind going deeper and deeper in one direction, we do āsanas or some study to help us gain clarity. We then might see that we are not on the right path. Failing this, the mind will continue to take over. Some Theosophists have caught this notion when they say the mind is a very faithful servant but a cruel master. The mind is not the master but very often it behaves as if it were. Therefore, it is useful for us to do some things which give the puruṣa some scope to see. If we get into a groove, the mind takes over and the puruṣa becomes ineffective.

Question: If we see with clarity does it mean that the mind no longer exists? Is there only the puruṣa?

Response: Clarity means you see how the mind functions and are able to handle it. It is never a matter of destroying the mind. That is impossible. It is control over the mind. We know our weaknesses, we know our strengths. We know what will lead us into more or less duḥkha. This is clarity. This is why we use the word viveka, "to see both sides." We are able to see what we are and what we are not. When we used the word asmitā, we defined it as ego. Asmitā is also a state where puruṣa and citta are mixed up and often form a unit within us. That is why there continues to be different interpretations of puruṣa and citta. When the puruṣa and the citta can be separated, we have viveka, the ability to see both sides.

In our consideration of duḥkha, one might ask, "What is to be done with duḥkha?" Though we appreciate that something must be done about duḥkha, the only duḥkha that matters is that which is about to come. Things that have happened or are happening must be accepted. Tomorrow's duḥkha can be avoided. We anticipate and then take preventative measures. This very important process is the only way we can actually avoid duḥkha in life. The whole of yoga is an attempt to do this. We know duḥkha is coming as long as avidyā is prevalent. The only origin of duḥkha is avidyā.

Question: Is there any concern with the past, as in psychotherapy, to understand duḥkha?

Response: Like going back to old memories?

Question: Yes, in order to understand?

Response: Take the example of a man who realizes

that he is in a groove. That groove is called saṃskāra. Saṃskāra is the total of all our actions that condition us to act in one way. Kara comes from the root kṛ which means "to do" or "to act." Sam means "complete, accumulated." Saṃskāra may be either positive or negative. We try to create a new positive saṃskāra, not reinforce the old, negative. The person who realizes he is in a groove should attempt to get out of it.

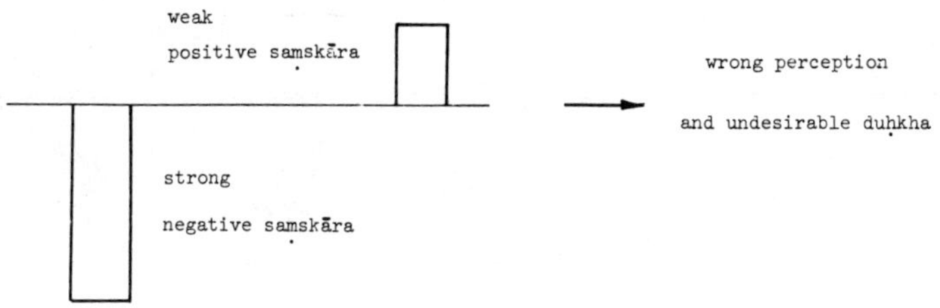

Fig. 40

Question: Must we recognize all the aspects of saṃskāra before we can create new?

Response: To see the problem is the first step. The next is to understand why we are getting duḥkha. What is its origin? Gradually we learn and once we know, we can conquer it. We have to create a new saṃskāra that is not negative but positive. If this new saṃskāra is powerful, the old one causing duḥkha will have no effect. We, in a way, start a whole new life. As the new ways become stronger, the old ways become ineffective.

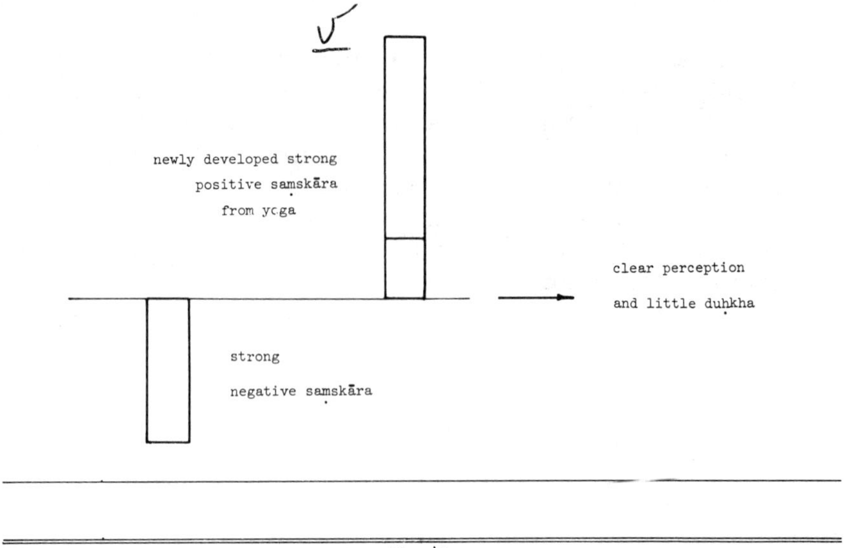

Fig. 41

Question: Is it important to understand the origins of our old negative saṃskāra?

Response: Sometimes this can be helpful, since there are many strengths of saṃskāra. It is only the strong, very influential ones that really bother us. While the weaker ones may support the strong, it is these that bring us our problems. Further, we might act in a way we thought was right and yet our actions result in trouble. When we have a quiet mind, inquiry into why our actions gave us trouble helps us to be more careful the next time. Also, the concept of pratipakṣa that we talked about earlier will be helpful. If we have to act, it is good to withdraw from that action and look at it again, afresh. In that way an understanding of saṃskāra can help.

Question: You said that yoga attempts to build positive saṃskāra and to render the negative ones ineffective. Don't we eventually have to get rid of the positive saṃskāra also?

Response: That is the next step, and it is one that can be taken in time. The *Yoga Sūtra* tells us that we should create powerful new *saṃskāra* to cause the old to disappear. Then it tells us, don't stop there but go on until there is no *saṃskāra*. Let us concern ourselves with only the first step now.

Question: Could a new *saṃskāra* bring *avidyā*?

Response: If the new *saṃskāra* is negative, there is *avidyā* while a positive *saṃskāra* means there is no *avidyā*. It is possible by practicing yoga to gradually reduce some old negative *saṃskāra*. Should we stop our practice and the old *saṃskāra* were again to take over, it would mean that the new positive *saṃskāra* was not powerful enough to make the old ineffective. This could be because we faced hurdles in strengthening the positive *saṃskāra*. A few of these might be disease, heaviness, doubts or hastiness. There is another problem. When we begin some of our practices we become healthier. Our senses behave better and because of this we become distracted. For example, we want to climb a hill to visit a temple. On the way we see a beautiful cashew grove. We stop to eat and we keep eating until we get sick. It is then impossible to go on to the temple. Similarly, when we do yoga, we develop increased sensitivity. If we become preoccupied with this sensitivity we might increase *avidyā*. Some people who practice yoga develop such a good physical condition that this becomes their only concern. If we carefully observe our actions, we will not have this problem.

Let me introduce another concept that relates to why we have *avidyā*. In this world we have two things: *puruṣa* and *prakṛti*. There is a question of whether there is only one *puruṣa* or many, but this will be covered later. Actually the term used in the *Yoga Sūtra* for *puruṣa* is *draṣṭṛ*; for *prakṛti*, *dṛśya*. *Draṣṭṛ* is the seer, that which sees; *dṛśya* is that which is seen. *Avidyā* exists when these two get mixed up. When the distinction between them is missing, it is known as *saṃyoga*. At that moment the seed for *duḥkha* is sown. While I will explain *puruṣa* and prakṛti more fully later, this diagram might help us to see that everything other than puruṣa is prakṛti. Everything that is observable, the mind, senses, body, etc. is prakṛti.

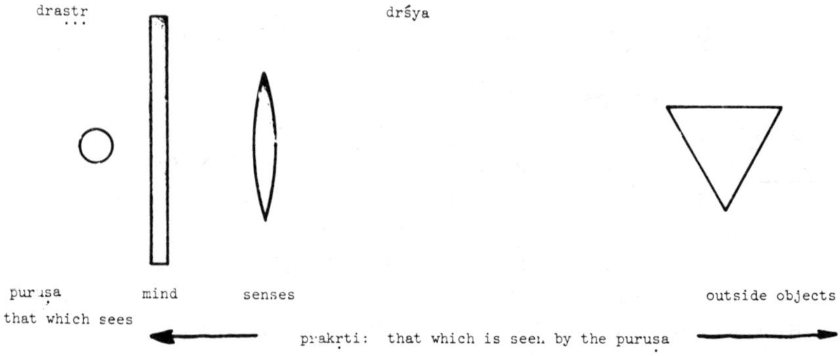

puruṣa and prakṛti

Fig. 42

Question: Is there a difference between saṃyoga and asmitā?

Response: Yes. One of the expressions of saṃyoga is asmitā. Asmitā is when the seer (cit) and the mind (citta) are associated, mixed up and held in an inseparable notion of I-ness. The mind is basically an instrument of perception and cit is the perceiver. The mind has a characteristic of change while cit does not. This association of two distinct entities often leads to problems.

Question: Along the same lines, what is the difference between saṃyoga and avidyā?

Response: They are not different. It is just one more way of looking at it. There is a sūtra that states avidyā is the taking of bad for good or good for bad, the changing as unchanging and the unchanging as changing.

This is the same as saṃyoga but in different terms.

Question: Would you say that a person would experience duḥkha if he were not seeking clarity?

Response: We are always experiencing duḥkha even though some of us might not be seeking clarity.

Question: What about someone who always thinks he is right, who always says "this doesn't bother me," meaning duḥkha doesn't bother him.

Response: When somebody says "this doesn't bother me," he is already bothered. The more we try to understand things, the more we can learn to anticipate duḥkha. Otherwise, we become trapped by duḥkha itself, a very sad condition.

VI

Theory

PURUṢA AND PRAKṚTI

To review--I began with several definitions of the word yoga. I mentioned that anyone can become involved in this study from any starting point or point of view; that there are no preconditions nor binding beliefs required, nor will particular religious beliefs interfere with practice. Yoga is a process to better ourselves. I next explained that there is a cover on the mind called avidyā that causes us to err in action. I noted that the different expressions of avidyā, the "I-thing," desire, dislike, and fear are sometimes weak and sometimes strong. Many of our actions come from this avidyā and lead us into other similar actions until we become conditioned. Yoga brings about a new process to reduce this conditioning. The concept of duḥkha was discussed. It comes from avidyā and disturbs the mind. The aim of yoga is to change the quality of action to avoid the duḥkha yet to come. I then introduced the concepts of puruṣa and prakṛti as being the two things that together make up this world. Prakṛti is "matter" that exists but is constantly changing. Puruṣa is something in the center of us that sees and does not change. It is the mixing (saṃyoga) of these two that brings about a disturbance of the mind.

Question: You said that in order to eliminate duḥkha we try to strike at the substance of avidyā. That seems a rather simplistic explanation for the way things actually work. Could you expand or elaborate on this?

Response: That which is required to avoid duḥkha is a different state of mind. This is why yoga places so much emphasis on the mind. Although there are hundreds of definitions of yoga, the most important one is to bring about a change in the quality of the mind. This means a change in its behavior, how it functions, how it perceives. Yoga attempts to bring about this change so that we can foresee something well in advance. This is wisdom. If we have yellow caution signals, we have time to find a solution. We create a condition by which the mind can see clearly, well in advance, and much more. This state of clarity will tell us whether to proceed with an action or to change, stop or wait. In this way we can avoid duḥkha. Experience will teach us to recognize duḥkha. Once we know what it is, we will be able to anticipate it before it is experienced and then try to avoid it. How we avoid it depends upon particular circumstances. There are no ready solutions to avoid or mitigate the various types of duḥkha. Instead, we try to develop a state of mind that will find appropriate answers. Those answers, not already formed, come with clarity of mind. It is like a clean mirror; even with a small amount of light, the reflection is automatic. When the mirror is dirty, there is no reflection even though the light is always present. The variable factor is the dirt or avidyā. Yoga is an attempt to remove this cover of avidyā.

Question: You said that wisdom is the result of clarity of mind. If avidyā and its effects are not continually present, do we all experience this wisdom or clarity from time to time?

Response: Yes. Even if we have not done anything in life to encourage it, clarity can come once in a while. Some people say it is divine grace, some say it is chance. The important thing is that we seek it, recognize it, and strive toward it. Yoga offers many suggestions about movement toward it.

Question: Why is it that often, even when we know certain actions will cause us duḥkha, it is more difficult to do the right thing than to act in a way we know we will regret?

Response: Even when some things are good, we cannot prompt ourselves to do them even by will. Some people try forcibly to restrain themselves from doing certain things. This will never work because the activity of forcing, constraining, and struggling tends to become a distraction. We become so involved in the negative action that we never progress. For example, some people know that smoking is harmful, and not just because the Surgeon General has said so. Someone might smoke sixty cigarettes a day, and he might understand intellectually that he should not smoke, but he cannot stop. Nobody smokes because they like the idea of inhaling tar and nicotine. There is some other reason; habit, of course, nervousness, perhaps. If such a person forces himself to stop smoking, he might suffer more than if he had continued. Instead, something must happen to such a person that will tell him, "Look here, I can do without cigarettes." Ideally, when we move into the practice of yoga, we begin to develop a process that stops the detrimental. This stopping is not caused directly--we don't stop the bad, it stops.

Let us turn to a fuller discussion of the concept of prakṛti. According to yoga teachings, the world is made up of only two things. One is the puruṣa, that which sees, but is sometimes prevented from seeing clearly by avidyā. The Yoga Sūtra uses the word draṣṭṛ for seer or observer. That which is seen by draṣṭṛ is dṛśya. The process of seeing starts in the mind. We think and we know that we are thinking, so we are able to see not only the outside but also the functions of the mind. Next the senses function as the instruments of perception. Finally there exist the objects of perception, all that is seen, the whole outside world. This whole process is not one of distinct events; they are interrelated. In fact, all things that fall in the realm of the seen were created from the same source. In the beginning this common source, called pradhāna, had no relation with the puruṣa. When the puruṣa came in contact with pradhāna it was as if a germ sprouted. This germ, prakṛti, multiplied and the material world evolved. First came mahat, the great principle. After mahat came ahaṃkāra, the "sense of I." From ahaṃkāra came the tanmātras and the indriyas. The tanmātras are the characteristics of sound, touch, form, taste, and smell. They were created in this order--out of sound came touch, out of touch came form, etc., moving from the subtlest to the grossest. The indriyas include, besides the mind, the senses of perception and action. Those of perception are hearing, feeling, seeing, tasting, and smelling; those of action are vocal, manual, locomotion, evacuation, and procreation. From the tanmātras came the bhūtas or elements of space, air, light, water, and earth. Thus, there are eleven senses and five elements having various forms.

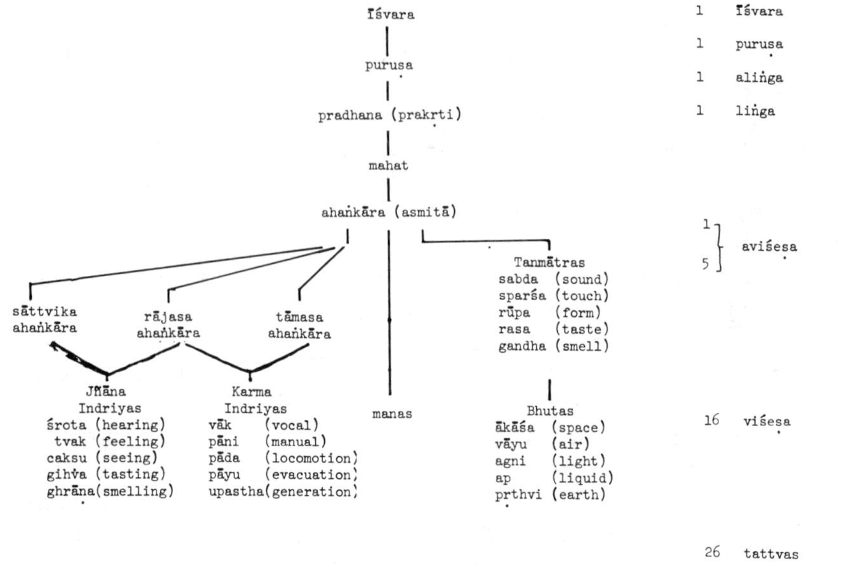

The 26 tattvas (principles)

Fig. 43

This is a brief and incomplete summary of the theory of evolution set forth by the yoga system. The world we see is the combination of all these things and because these things evolve successively one to another, they are interrelated. What happens in the outside world influences us and what happens in us influences our relation to the outside world. As an example, there are people who are not able to sleep during a full moon. There are others who become disturbed during an eclipse. The whole concept of astrology infers that a relationship exists between all things because they all come from the same root. The eleven senses and five elements form the components of what is perceived.

There is no source in yoga that explains whether the origin of primal pradhāna or puruṣa was from the Lord or simply there. There is no description of the puruṣa other than that it sees and only through the mind. We cannot do anything about the quality of puruṣa; it is constant. Our practice in yoga is to effect a change in the quality of the mind so that the observation of the puruṣa, which is through the mind, is not distorted. When the mind thinks it is see-

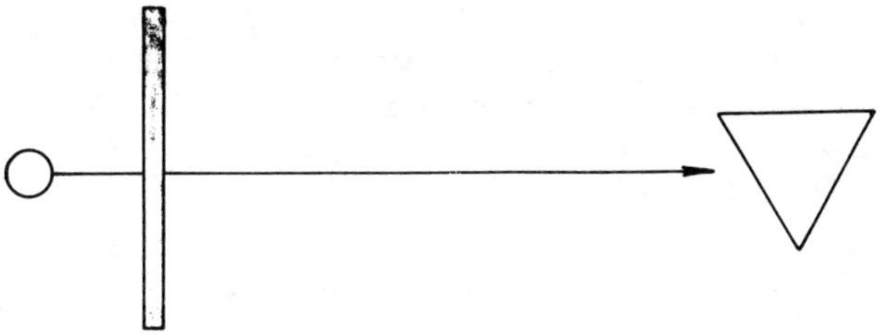

observation is by the puruṣa but through the mind

Fig. 44

ing rather than the puruṣa there is avidyā, and this is the beginning of duḥkha. The mind is an accumulation of actions and the memories of actions. This conditions us to act as we have been acting. In so doing, we cannot detect that things are changing and therefore, our actions might go wrong. It is important that we remember the distinct and different characteristics of puruṣa and prakṛti. Puruṣa is unchanging; prakṛti changes, and mind is a part of prakṛti.

Question: Does that mean the puruṣa has no existence independent of the mind? If there is severe brain damage is there a puruṣa?

Response: The best way to understand puruṣa is to think of it as that which is absent in a dead body. In death the puruṣa vanishes. The body, brain, and senses are still there but are lifeless because puruṣa is absent. There is no other way to describe the puruṣa. It cannot be seen by the mind. We only know it is present because sometimes we have clarity. It is the constant witness to all our action. The basic concept is that puruṣa is an active witness uninfluenced by that which it sees. Since it can only see through the mind, it can only see correctly if the mind is clear. As human beings, we cannot think of an independent existence of puruṣa and prakṛti. In man, the two are always related. Why has there been a confusion of puruṣa and prakṛti? According to the Yoga Sūtra, the whole saṃyoga or confusion between prakṛti and puruṣa is in our life so that those who are inclined to seek clarity can learn the distinction between correct and incorrect understanding. In this sense, yoga is optimistic; we move through our recognition of problems and confusion into a quest for clarity.

Because some of us might seek solutions to problems and in so doing gain some degree of clarity does not mean that puruṣa will see more clearly in others. This proves that there are different puruṣas, all in their own "cities." Other philosophical systems say there is only one puruṣa; however, if one man gains freedom from his problems, it does not mean all have freedom. Thus, there are different puruṣas, though only one prakṛti. There is only one common universe for us. The contact between one puruṣa and prakṛti is different; therefore, the way we see things, our bodies, our senses, our conditioning, all are different.

Question: Does the puruṣa generate that which is out in the world?

Response: Yes. Observation only happens if there is energy and an inclination on the part of puruṣa to go out, as it were, and bring back an impression. This is different from modern physics where there must be light in order for an image to come to the eye. Even if there is a light and an object for it to fall upon something must provoke us to see, to listen, to think. That which triggers this action comes from the puruṣa, not from the outside. Often external things try to provoke and yet we do not react. This demonstrates that all action must come from puruṣa. Further, man does not exist without puruṣa.

Question: How does this relationship with the puruṣa come about?

Response: Different schools have different opinions about this. Some say it is līlā or the "sport" of the Lord. Others believe that in the beginning there was only one thing that said, "let me multiply." Still others say it was chance. Any stand we take will be speculative. It is as difficult to explain as death. How can we know? We develop many theories because of our discursive intellects. Who can experience the beginning of the world? We talk about death when we are alive. I can repeat the theories but I don't really know.

Question: Does puruṣa have the potential to explain things like what happens after death?

Response: There is no death for the puruṣa because there is no change for it, and what is death but change. Since the puruṣa has no death, even if it were able to speak, it might lack the experience to explain. What explains is our intelligence based on our memory. Any explanation we give for actions that we have or have not experienced comes from the mind because words emanate from there. Words do not emanate from puruṣa.

Question: Does puruṣa act?

Response: Its action is that it sees. It is like a dry cell. A dry cell has potential energy if put in the proper position to give power. Puruṣa acts in that it gives energy for action. It does not act in the sense of walking or talking. All actions that we are able to see come from prakṛti but the source for these actions, the energy, comes from puruṣa.

Question: Does the decision making process, which occurs before our action, take place in the mind with the puruṣa as simply an observer?

Response: Yes. As the mind changes, action becomes different. The puruṣa stays the same. Change in action is due to change in the state of mind. We might argue with someone and the next day feel very sorry. We are the same person, only our state of mind has changed.

Question: Does the puruṣa go into another form when we die?

Response: There are several theories. People who believe in something higher than us, the Lord, say different puruṣas are like different rivers. They have their own course of flow, their own direction, and their own quality; but they all join in the sea. What happens to the river? Everything becomes the ocean. Others who use the metaphor of the great ocean to represent the Lord say that puruṣa is a river. When we are free from the body it is as though the river has joined the sea. Since this is said to occur after death it is difficult for me to confirm. It is mostly speculation. Still others say that there is only one puruṣa. They say that the apparent differences are like scratches on a piece of glass. When we die, the scratch vanishes, or our individual identity no longer exists. What we thought of as different puruṣas were just "scratches" on the great puruṣa. There are quite a few theories on this and you can accept whichever you like.

Question: Is there an explanation for how the mind can bring about changes in itself?

Response: If we are constantly acting in one way, we tend to continue to act that way. How can we ever change? It is difficult to say we changed because we practiced yoga, Zen or any other system. There are those who change as the result of practice and those who never change in spite of practice. In other words, change is not the direct or immediate result of work in yoga or any other practice. We never know. What we do know is that somehow the qualities of heaviness and "dancing" in the mind are eliminated. Some people insist that we only change through the grace of God (Īśvara). I don't know. It could be just the quality of the mind or it could be divine grace. The point is that good action does not always result from a specific, particular action. Something fundamental must happen at the right moment, something so strong and so striking that we really want to stop, think and change our course of action. After that happens, little by little we progress. There begins a change in the quality of our action. The new positive saṃskāra becomes stronger and the mind will stay clear.

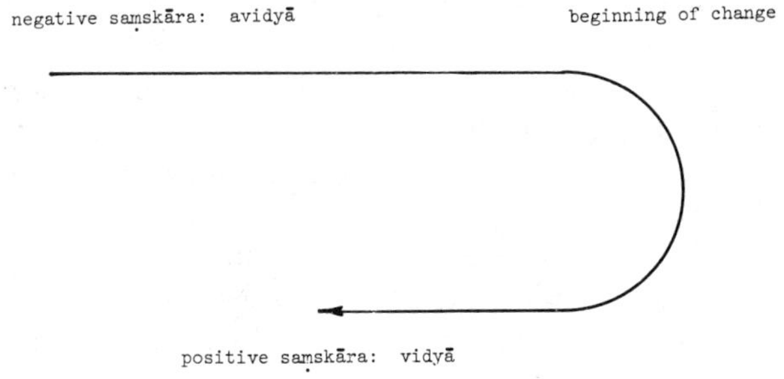

the change from negative to positive saṃskāra

Fig. 45

Question: Clarity is a state of mind or quality of mind. I don't understand the need for the concept of puruṣa?

Response: Your question is if clarity is in the mind,

why should there be puruṣa? Who is going to know if there is or is not clarity? We need an element outside the mind to witness clarity. That is why puruṣa is important. It is like we are a part of a flowing river. Sometimes the river goes quickly, sometimes the river goes slowly, and sometimes it meets the ocean. Unless we have something in us that can feel the speed of movement, we cannot say whether the river is flowing or not.

Question: So the mind isn't able to observe itself?

Response: The mind is not able to observe its own changes. Something else observes those changes.

Question: And puruṣa always works through the mind?

Response: Yes. That is why we described puruṣa as a witness as well as the source of action. As a source of action, it is like an electric garage door transmitter. The source of action is the transmitter but what moves is the garage door. The puruṣa is like the transmitter and the mind like the garage door. So we need puruṣa as the source of action. We also need puruṣa as a witness, as a constant observer of the mind's functions. Finally, clarity is in the mind, but the experiential understanding is by the puruṣa. In the clear understanding there is peace. Someone asked me how we can know if clarity is from the puruṣa or just in the mind. When there is clarity, there is silence. When there is intellectual clarity we are happy, we are pleased but this might not last.

Our goal is to be free from duḥkha. We must recognize duḥkha, we must know it is caused by avidyā, we must understand that it can be avoided and, finally, that this is achieved hopefully by the practice of yoga, whether it be āsana, prāṇāyāma or reflection.

VII

Practice

IMPROVISATION IN ĀSANA

At this stage in our introductory practice of yoga, let us discuss improvisation in āsana. As we continue āsana practice using a variety of postures and breathing in a planned sequence, somehow we get used to the routine. Gradually our attention to our practice decreases. People often say they get bored doing the same postures over and over again. This, then, is a reason for improvisation, to bring a new quality of attention and a sense of discovery to our practice. By attention we mean to be present in what we are doing and to feel what we are doing. By sense of discovery we mean to see something we did not see before. Unless we improvise, rather than doing the same thing over and over again, this sense of discovery, so important in yoga, will be missing.

There is an important effect of attention and discovery in āsana practice. Before we begin our daily āsana practice we might have quite a few things on our minds, that is, we might be in a distracted state of mind. Actually, unless we are either asleep or completely involved in a favored activity, the mind always jumps from one thing to another. If we are doing āsanas and the mind continues to wander, we are not doing the āsanas, only our bodies are doing them. To reduce this movement so that the mind is focused on what we are doing, improvisation is necessary. Unfortunately, once we get into a habit of doing postures the mind can wander even while we are doing them. We may end up feeling supple, our pulse rate will come down, but this is not complete practice. There is a need to focus the mind and this happens automatically when there is attention and discovery.

Another reason for improvisation is physical improvement. We can't deny that when we begin a program we would like to get something specific out of it, to achieve some special result. Such results, strengthening the back, reducing weight, or freeing us from asthma are achieved through improvisation. For example, a man who has one shoulder that is much stiffer than the other might do some modified āsanas by which that stiffness might be reduced. At the same time this improvisation might be enjoyable. His interest and attention on what he is doing might increase because he knows that he is doing it for the sake of his shoulder. Improvisation can help solve a physical problem and can also help us avoid duḥkha. What might be good or possible for one person can have a negative effect on another. We must carefully consider a person's condition and then improvise so that he or she might gain something without getting into trouble. That explains why, in our practice classes, we suggest different things for different people.

One last reason for improvisation is efficiency, to get the maximum results through minimum effort, to do less to get more. Improvisation can save us time and also obtain better results. If we know how to do a posture in an intelligent way, we can achieve the most beneficial results from that posture. This is efficiency. These, then, are the reasons for improvisation: attention, discovery, focus, special results, efficiency.

The easiest way to improvise is to modify the āsana. For example, uttānāsana can be modified in many ways. If we want to use the posture to increase the effect on our legs rather than the back, we bend forward and place our palms on the floor. Keeping the palms on the floor, we try to stretch our legs and straighten our backs on inhalation. Suppose we want to use uttānāsana to strengthen the back. We bend forward as far as we can and then come up half-way. In this case we use the back muscles to work against gravity. If we want to use uttānāsana to help straighten stooping shoulders, we interlock our fingers behind our backs, palms out, and bend forward raising the arms. We can also use uttānāsana for people with stiff ankles. People performing ballet sometimes have this problem. In this case we use some padding under our heels. This takes the strain off our ankles and makes bending forward easier. If, on the other hand, we want to

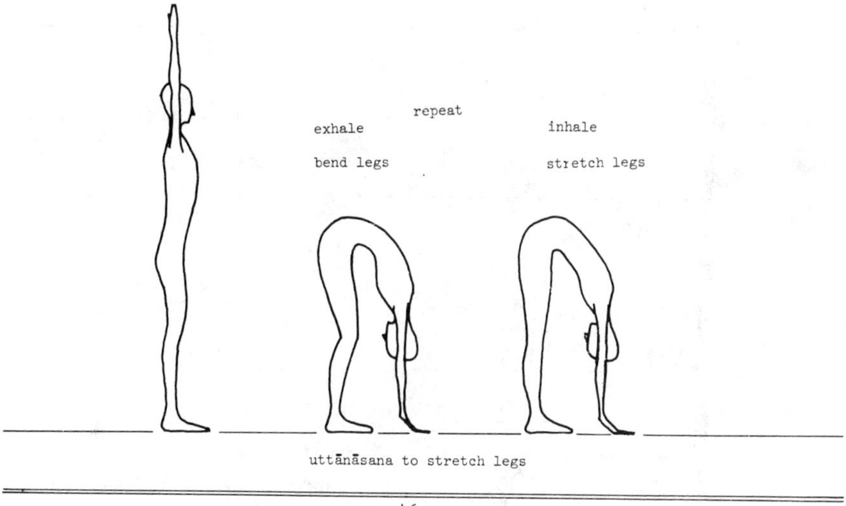

Fig. 46

stretch the ankles, we put the padding under our toes. It is all the same āsana but the attention is placed on different areas or needs. In this way we can do many variations. These variations are not just for people with particular problems. They help give everyone a sense of discovery. If we modify a posture we can see how it affects the different parts of our bodies.

Another way of improvising is to modify our breathing. For example, we can control the breath to make an inhalation equal to an exhalation. If this is our plan, from the moment we start the posture our attention must be upon breathing. We can make the time of inhalation equal to the time of holding the breath or we can make the time of exhalation equal to that of holding the breath, or any number of variations.

We have noted that one way of improvising is to vary the way we do a posture. Any posture can be done in

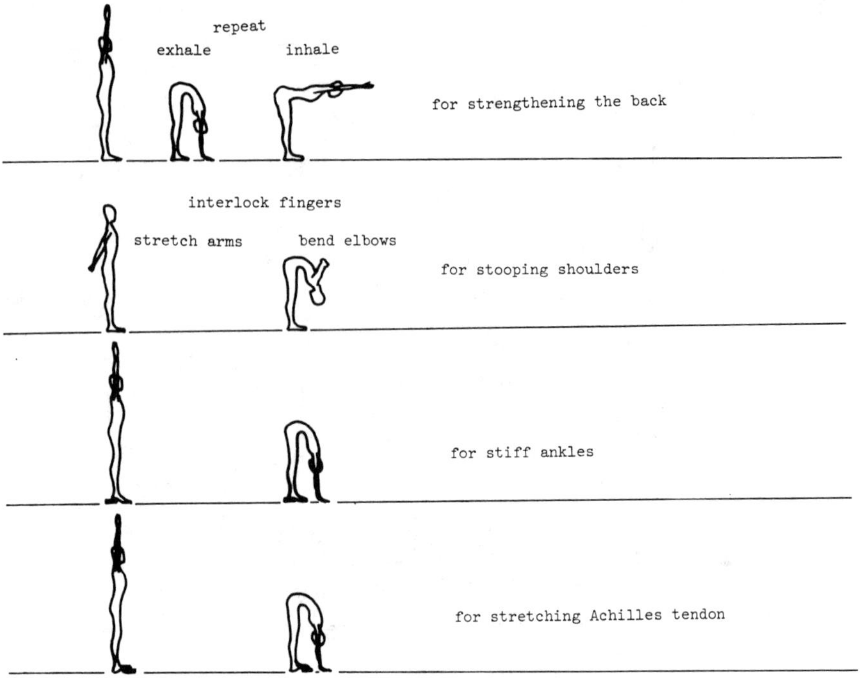

variations of uttānāsana

Fig. 47

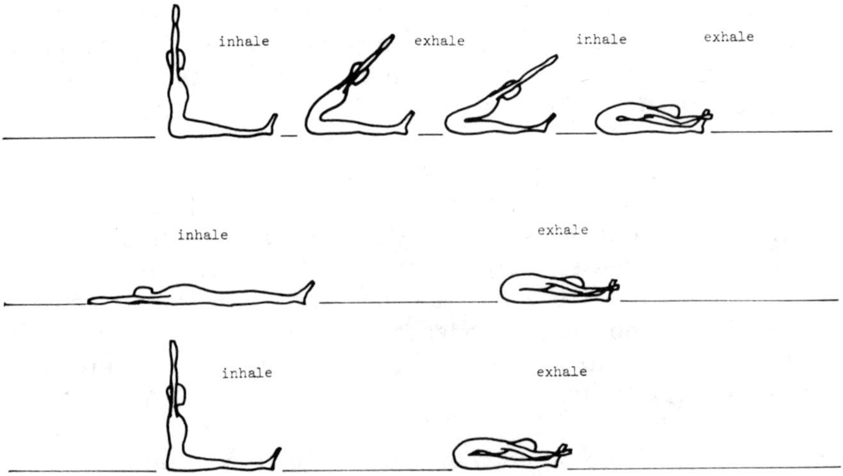

variations of paścimatānāsana

Fig. 48

many ways. For example, paścimatānāsana can begin in several ways, sitting up or lying down. We can also use a different technique in the same posture. It is practiced in two steps. On the first exhalation we bend forward halfway, stay and arch the back on inhalation and on the next exhalation go on down.

The way we do a posture will determine its effect. Also, what we do before a posture can determine where the action will be felt. Often people say they feel nothing in a posture. They want to feel something in their muscles and they think nothing is happening. To assist people in learning to feel, we can change a technique or begin with an opposite posture before the main movement. This will assure them that something is really happening.

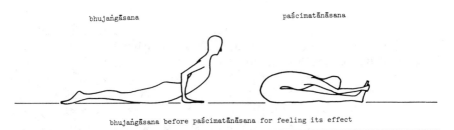

bhujaṅgāsana before paścimatānāsana for feeling its effect

Fig. 49

One more way of improvisation is to shift our attention during a posture to different parts of the body, as in the following example, bhujaṅgāsana:

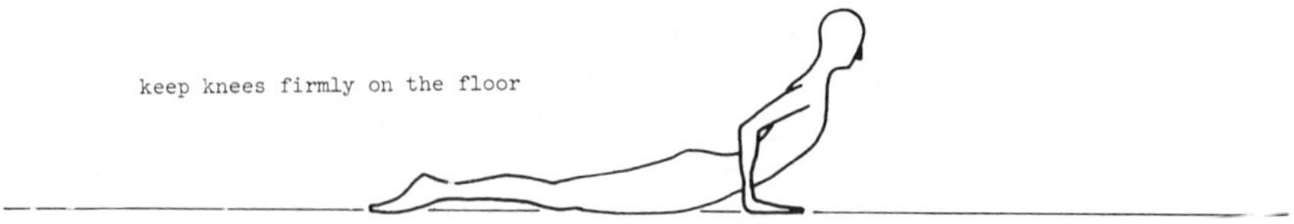
arch the back during each inhalation
keep knees firmly on the floor
bhujaṅgāsana keeping feet and knees on the floor

Fig. 50

We can focus our attention upon our knees to be sure they stay on the floor. To achieve this, it might be necessary to add some special action for the knees, such as pressing them down. Normally when beginners try this posture, as they go up, their legs rise slightly off the floor. If we try to keep the legs down, the whole feeling is different. Thus, this shifting of attention brings added quality to our āsana practice. We can also raise the spine in coordination with the breath and focus our attention upon the area we are raising. Yet another possibility is to hold a book between our hands with fingers flat. Our normal tendency is to curl the fingers but when we do bhujaṅgāsana with a book we feel more of a reaction in our arms, shoulders, and upper back than in the lower back. By using an external means, such as the book, we also bring a new quality of attention.

Śalabhāsana (locust posture, prone with upper body and legs raised) provides another example. This posture is like bhujaṅgāsana except that we also lift our legs. Under normal conditions, some people might think this is

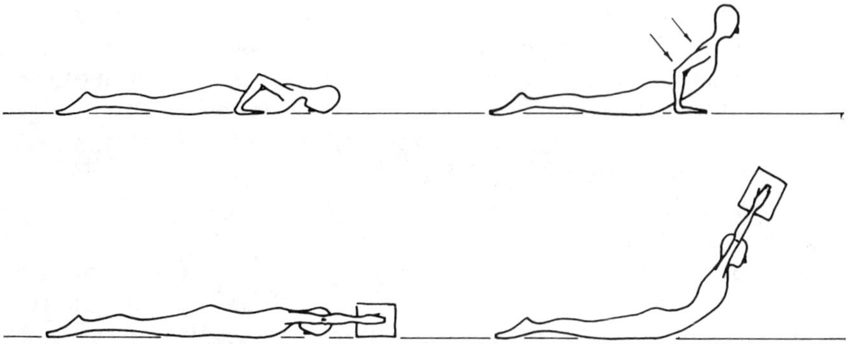

to bring attention to arms, shoulders and upper back: hold a book

Fig. 51

such a simple posture, but with a book or a towel between the knees, it is not really so simple or easy. We find it very difficult to keep the knees together when bending backward. The legs spread more the higher we lift them. With

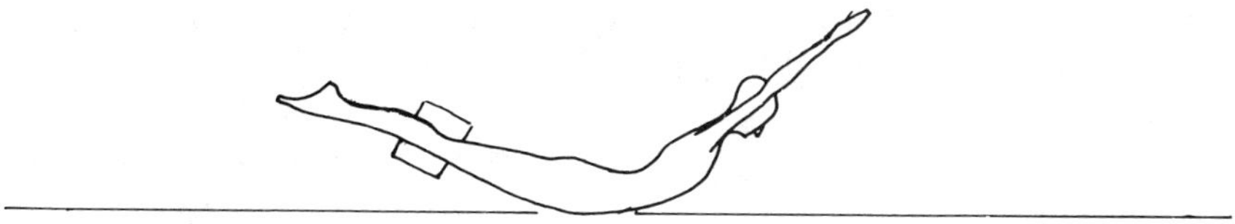

śalabhāsana with a book held between knees

Fig. 52

a book held gently between the knees, many people can hardly lift their legs. For the first time they feel the effects of the posture at certain places on their backs.

Thus we use improvisation to bring something new and useful into the practice of _āsana_. Therefore, if one of you is asked to do an _āsana_ with legs straight and another to do that same _āsana_ with legs bent, please don't think you are winning or losing a contest. Since this is not dance, form is not important. What is important when doing an _āsana_ is the experience that happens at the moment. Some of you might be told to bend your knees, others to hold or not hold your breath after inhalation, and others to hold or not hold after exhalation. These individual variations are necessary because we must respect the reality of our individual conditions.

Question: Could you explain the various ways of using the breath in _āsana_ movement?

Response: There are two ways that we do postures. We can do a posture dynamically, that is, to repeat the movement, and we can do it statically, that is, to stay in a posture. Within these types, the following variations are possible:

(1) Free breathing. Inhalation and exhalation as long as possible using the throat restriction.

(2) Making the inhalation equal to the exhalation. In some postures this will be easy; however very often the length of exhalation or inhalation, depending upon the movement, will be different.

(3) Making the exhalation twice the length of the inhalation.

(4) Holding the breath after inhalation.

(5) Holding the breath after exhalation.

(6) Holding the breath after both inhalation and exhalation.

(7) Inhalation, exhalation, then doing a pose while holding the breath. Usually we do certain movements in coordination with either inhalation or exhalation. Sometimes, however, it is useful to do movements while holding after exhalation to help us warm up, particularly if it is cold. For example, inhale, exhale, and then while holding the breath do utkaṭāsana.

squat during exhalation
squat after exhalation, holding the breath throughout

utkaṭāsana   movement on different breathing rhythms

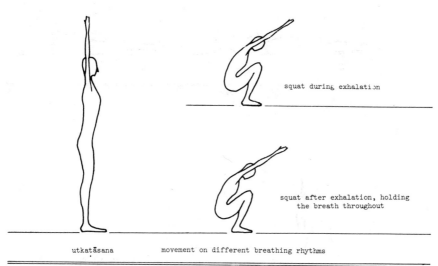

Fig. 53

(8) Another interesting way to change the breathing is to reverse the normal breath movement pattern. For example, when we do bhujaṅgāsana, rather than raising during inhalation, we raise during exhalation. Often we use the abdomen to push ourselves up in this posture rather than the back muscles. If we go up on inhalation the abdomen can push against the floor. Often we resort to going up on exhale to make the posture milder for people who have had abdominal surgery. Following such surgery, even after two or three weeks, it is better that all movements

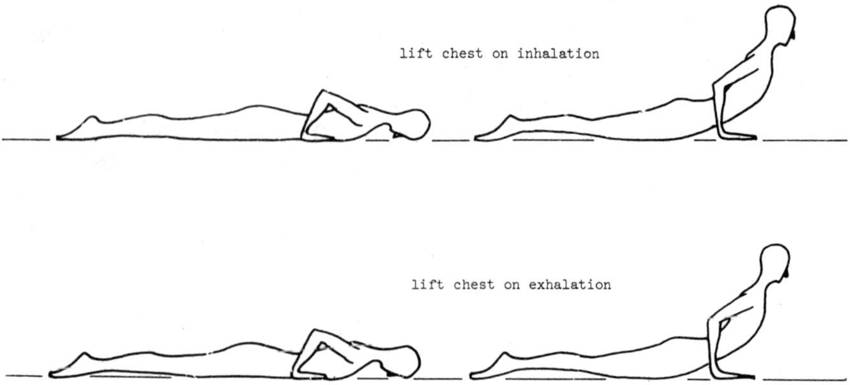
lift chest on inhalation
lift chest on exhalation

bhujaṅgāsana using different rhythms of breathing

Fig. 54

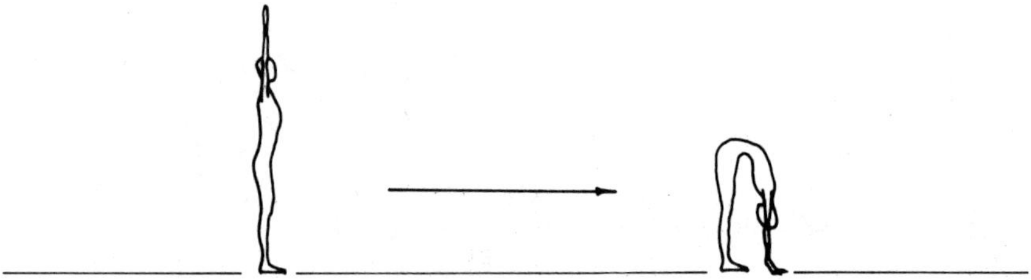

	starting posture	movement	final posture
1	inhale	during exhalation	stay a few breaths
2	inhale-hold breath	during exhalation	do not stay
3	inhale exhale	after exhalation	hold posture a few seconds
4	stay a few breaths	during exhalation	stay a few breaths
5	inhale- hold breath	during exhalation	hold posture a few seconds

various ways of doing uttānāsana

Fig. 55a

be done on exhalation lest the stitches come out.

Question: Wouldn't trying all kinds of improvisation at random inhibit progress? Doesn't a certain amount of attention and discovery come with steady, continued practice?

Response: Improvisation should not be done at random. Perhaps a certain amount of random experimentation is useful to understand the concept of improvisation. Generally, improvisation should be done only when it is warranted. When we are doing a posture and we find it monotonous, we should improvise. Otherwise, the point of your question is correct. We will be more distracted than helped by improvisation. We can only begin to improvise after we begin to understand the various postures. We do not suggest improvisation for the sake of improvisation. We do it when we need help to develop or to sustain attention, or as an aid to a particular physical need. This is particularly important in group classes. When a particular posture is introduced everyone cannot be expected to do it the same way. It is necessary to improvise to avoid doing harm to any given individual. One of my students had sprained a shoulder in some game. In class we were doing a posture and everybody tried to keep their arms straight. Trying to straighten his arms gave him pain so I instructed him to bend his arms at the elbows. Improvise when there is a physical need or when you are trying to bring back a certain quality to the āsana.

Question: You gave us some variations in uttānāsana which were useful for different problems. Are there any similar principles about what type of breathing is useful at different times?

Response: Yes. Normally, we breathe in a certain way, beginning in the chest and moving to the abdomen. Inhalation involves the upper portion of the torso, the chest and diaphragm, as well as the spine. Exhalation, in terms of movement, involves the contraction of the abdomen. If we want to increase the effect on the chest we concentrate on the inhalation. If we want to increase the effect on the

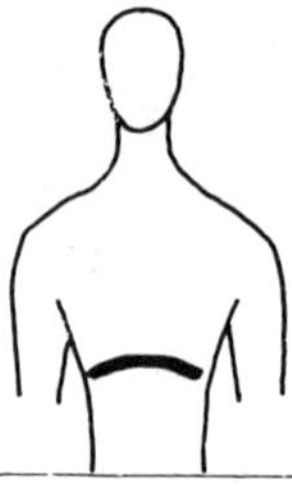
chest
abdomen
for working on chest emphasize inhaling and hold after inhalation
for working on abdomen, emphasize exhaling and hold after exhalation

adapting breathing to vary the effect of the āsana

Fig. 55b

abdomen or stomach, we concentrate on exhalation. I once had a student who had been a very powerful gymnast. He was still very strong with an unusually low pulse rate, just 40; however, he could hardly breathe! His inhalation and exhalation couldn't have been longer than three or four seconds because he had given up his gymnastics and his muscles had become very hard. They had lost their elasticity and resilience, so he couldn't expand his chest. I had him use a free or untimed inhalation, holding the breath after inhalation, then free exhalation. Gradually, holding the breath began to stretch the intercostal muscles and those that cover the chest. As they became looser he was able to breathe more slowly, to extend the time of inhalation and exhalation. We use the inhalation followed by holding the breath in order to increase the muscular flexibility and breathing capacity of the chest region. We are not talking about the heart, only the chest. When there are problems in the abdomen like constipation or overweight, we focus upon that area by concentrating upon exhalation and holding the breath after exhalation. About the heart--if someone has a weak heart we never hold the breath after inhalation because it builds up pressure and increases anxiety. For such persons, we usually establish an inhalation/exhalation ratio of one to two. If someone has a pulse rate of 92-100, even from little exercise, it is always better to have them concentrate upon long exhalations even when doing āsanas.

Imagine we want to use breathing in āsanas to focus on the upper back. We select postures that emphasize that area and at the same time we hold our breath after inhalation. The opposite is true if we want to emphasize the lower back. There is a method to improvisation. Improvisation should not be used for its own sake. It has two purposes--to bring attention and to fulfill a particular need.

We have briefly covered the definition of posture, breathing in posture, planning, the concepts of preparation and counterpose and why and how to improvise. Any questions?

Question: Is it possible to immediately follow or precede the practice of āsanas or prāṇāyāma with some other type of physical discipline or participation in a sport?

Response: Generally it is all right to move from yoga practice to other activities provided we rest in between. Moving from other exercises to āsanas presents problems. The whole attitude when we run or play such games as tennis is different from when we do āsanas. If we have just lost our tennis match we might be thinking of it while we are doing āsanas. We might not be present in our practice. Physiological problems could also arise. In some sports such as running, tennis, and skiing, muscles are always contracted. If we immediately try to do stretching or bending backward exercises we will develop cramps. If we must do āsanas after physical activities, take a long break. Without this, there is usually a problem of mental orientation and physiological readiness. We should avoid sandwiching any other activity into a planned sequence of āsana practice. If you want to do both āsanas and sports, try to do the āsanas before the sport or else provide a long break between the two.

Question: Is the same true of prāṇāyāma in relation to sports or vigorous exercise?

Response: Generally anything before prāṇāyāma is all right provided there is an adequate break for transition. It also depends on the sport. The whole state of mind is different in prāṇāyāma. Sports are often competitive. If we are going to engage in a competitive sport after prāṇāyāma, we must allow an adequate transition because this breathing practice makes us calm. We have to boost ourselves a little bit before we do vigorous exercise. Also in prāṇāyāma, generally we sit cross-legged. If we have done prāṇāyāma and then want to do a sport, do some standing āsanas as a transition to warm up the body and prepare the mind. On the other hand, a performer who might have stage fright will find that controlled breathing is very helpful. Since the problem is nervousness, a very relaxing type of prāṇāyāma calms the nerves.

Sometimes when we are exhausted after some physical activity, we can just lie down and do some simple breathing, such as free inhalation and long fixed exhalations. To use this as a means of bringing us back to a normal condition might be very useful.

Question: If in our āsana practice we are doing a lot of stretching exercises, for example those involving the legs, is it necessary to compensate by doing something to build up the muscles?

Response: I don't know how far we should go in building up the muscles. Some muscle action is required. A person who has had poliomyelitis might find it useful to modify postures in such a way as to affect the muscle tone of atrophied limbs. We can build muscles but there should be a limit. Too much muscle is a burden, unless we want to use it for a specific purpose such as weight lifting. There are cases, however, of people who have large torsos and very small legs. It can be quite tiring for them to hike or even to walk. For them, muscle building is necessary and they can use yoga for this. Some standing postures develop the legs, such as ardha utkaṭāsana (half

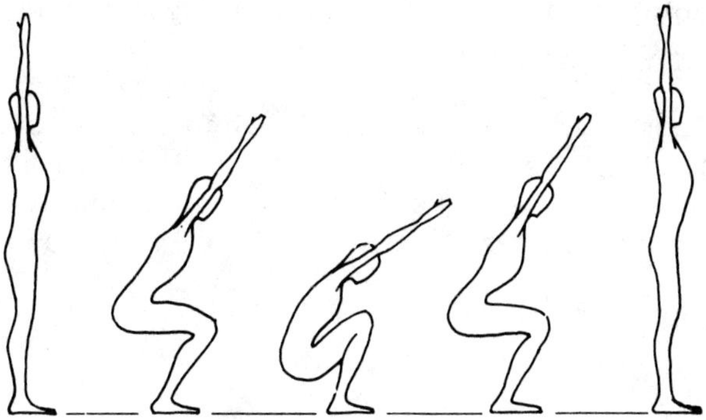

ardha utkaṭāsana to work on leg muscles

Fig. 56

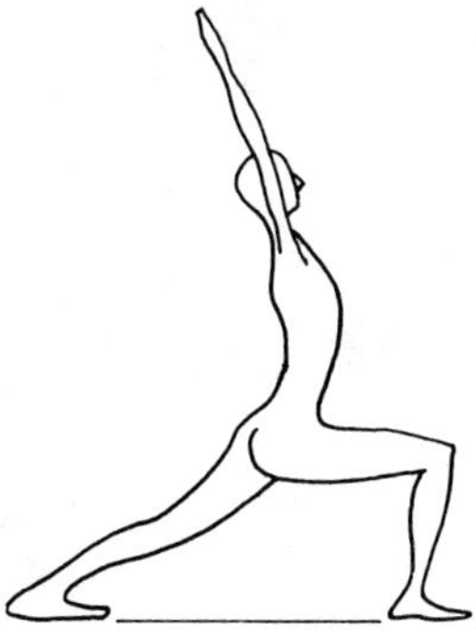

Vīrabhadrāsana

Fig. 57

squat). This posture is like weight lifting. Other postures like vīrabhadrāsana (standing, bending backward with one knee bent) will also help. The principle is--we must bring action to the area of the body we wish to improve.

Question: I find that if I do too much leg stretching without doing some kind of compensatory muscular activity, my legs bother me.

Response: That is exactly why we must use counterposes. It is also not a good idea to do an excessive amount of stretching. We must proceed gradually and use the necessary counterposes.

VIII

Theory

YAMA, NIYAMA AND ĀSANA--THE FIRST THREE AṄGAS OF YOGA

We have discussed avidyā and have noted the importance of reducing it to lessen duḥkha. We do this through movement from our present condition to a point where there is less duḥkha. Yoga does not offer us a specific method, in that, if we do this, such will happen. While there is an element of direct results from specific acts, this is by exception and not the general rule. Yoga also suggests that our attitude toward things can help in this movement toward reduced avidyā and freedom from duḥkha. The entire practice of yoga, as we are beginning to see, consists of certain attitudes, actions and their consequences.

Let us consider the attitudes yoga suggests we hold

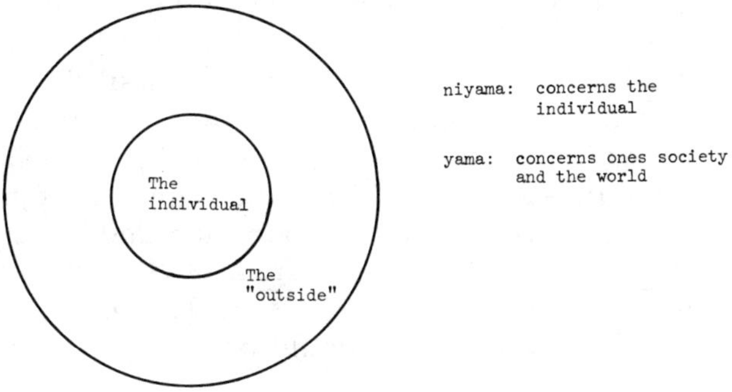
The
individual
The
"outside"
niyama: concerns the individual
yama: concerns ones society and the world

Yama and niyama: their context

Fig. 58

toward each other and ourselves. Attitudes toward "the outside" are called yamas and those toward "the inside," niyamas. These are the first two of eight limbs or aṅgas used in yoga. These two words have many meanings. Yama can mean discipline, restraints, etc., but attitude is a preferable definition. If we have a particular attitude, it may also be a discipline.

Patañjali's Yoga Sūtra considers five different attitudes (yamas) or relationships between an individual and "the outside." The first is ahiṃsā. While the word hiṃsā means injury, cruelty, etc., ahiṃsā means more than merely the absence of hiṃsā. It means kindness, consideration, etc. Ahiṃsā means "thoughtful consideration of people and things." We have to use a certain amount of judgment in this. It does not necessarily mean that we must not eat meat, catch fish, go to war, etc. While it may come to this, we must consider our circumstances and accordingly follow this concept of ahiṃsā, namely, to be considerate. Ahiṃsā not only means kindness to "the outside" but to ourselves as well. Suppose we are in a situation where only meat or fish is available. If we are vegetarians, should we allow ourselves to starve to death or should we eat what is available? On no account should we cause injury to ourselves if we think we still have things to do in life. What if we have responsibilities, such as a family? Shouldn't we eat whatever food is available to keep us fit and able to meet our responsibilities? Also, if I, a vegetarian, condemn others for eating meat, it would be a lack of consideration on my part just as much as if they insisted I eat meat. We must examine each circumstance with an attitude of consideration and kindness. This, then, is ahiṃsā. Finally, ahiṃsā is conditioned by duty. We have to do our duty. This could even mean that if our lives were threatened, it would be our duty to fight.

The next yama is called satya. The word satya means "to speak the truth." It is not always desirable to speak the truth, come what may. Speaking the truth is good, but not if it harms others. We must consider what we are going to say, how we are going to say it and how it will affect others. If speaking the truth will harm someone, it is best to keep quiet. Satya should never conflict with or work against ahiṃsā. The Mahābhārata, spoken by Dharmarāja, says "speak truth that is pleasant. Never speak truth that is not pleasant. Don't speak a lie, even if it is pleasant to hear. This is the eternal dharma."

The third yama is asteya. Steya means "to steal," asteya, the opposite. Simply put, asteya means "if we are in a situation where people trust us, we will not take advantage of them."

The next yama is brahmacarya. The word brahmacarya is composed of the root car, meaning "to move" and brahma meaning "truth." Brahmacarya is "to move in the direction of truth." It is often used to mean celibacy. However, it more specifically means that we must create a condition in our relationship to other beings and things that fosters understanding of the highest truths. If we move toward the understanding of truth and sensual pleasures get in the way, we must keep our direction and not become lost. Some people explain brahmacarya as continence, self restraint from sexual activity. If we do everything to help ourselves move toward truth, there arises some control over the ten organs of sense and action. This does not mean total abstinence. In fact, India holds the greatest respect for the gṛhastha or family man. Life is in four stages. They are the growing child, the brahmacāri or student seeking truth, the family man and, finally, the person who, having fulfilled a family obligation, strives to be free from all bondages. The family life is the most important. A sannyāsin or monk must beg for food. He must go to a family, a house where there is a wife and children to receive food. The Upaniṣads instruct the student who has finished his studies to get married and have children. Therefore, brahmacarya does not infer continence. It means responsibility so that gradually we move toward truth.

The last yama is aparigraha. Aparigraha means "hands off," "not to grasp." Parigraha is the opposite of the word dāna, which means "to give." In the way we use aparigraha it means "to receive exactly what is appropriate." I had a student who worked with me for some time.

Each month he paid me a fee for my teaching. At the end of the course he also presented to me a gift. Why should I receive a gift when I have already been paid for the work I have done? We must receive only what we deserve, otherwise it is exploitation. Also to receive undeserved recompense tends to create obligations and bondages.

The Yoga Sūtra describes what happens when these five attitudes become steadfast in a person. The more we develop kindness and consideration, that is, ahiṃsā, the more our presence engenders friendship.

Satya, as a yama, means "to speak the truth when and only when it is good for people." There is a beautiful episode in the Rāmāyaṇa about this. The monkey, Hanuman, goes to find the wife of Lord Rāma. At the end of his stay in Lanka he was caught and his tail was set afire causing him great suffering. Rāma's wife Sītā, seeing this, said, "Let the fire become cool." Immediately Hanuman exclaimed, "What is this? Why does the fire feel cool?" Sītā always spoke the truth, and, because of this, her words had this extraordinary power. For everyone who speaks the truth, there is no difference between what they do and what they say, and what they say, will be.

It is said that to a person with asteya all jewels will come. A person with asteya may not care for jewels; however, they will have access to everything that is precious in life.

If we do everything possible to move toward truth, brahmacarya, we will develop a capacity to go in that direction. The more we see the importance of this, the less we become involved in other activities. Naturally, we will need great vitality to pursue this course. The word used to describe this vitality is vīrya. Vīrya as used in the Yoga Sūtra is linked to the word śraddhā. Śraddhā means love or faith; we have an inspired passion to do something. The Yoga Sūtra states the more śraddhā present, the more vīrya we find we have. Obviously, we will have more strength to pursue our goal. In brahmacarya the more we seek truth, the more vitality we will have to do so.

Parigraha is more and more a movement toward materialism. The reduction of parigraha, that is, aparigraha, means we turn more inward. The less time we spend on having possessions, the more we have to investigate all that we call yoga. Therefore, we can find the answers more quickly. These, then, are our five attitudes as they relate to "the outside." Remarkable things can happen when we develop them.

It is important to emphasize that we do not start yoga by first doing ahiṃsā and when that is mastered, doing satya, etc. As we progress, seeking to better ourselves by any means, very gradually these things happen. An important usage of the word aṅga occurs in this context. Aṅga means a limb of the body. When we are born, every part of the body grows together. It is not that one arm grows and then a leg. In the same way, if we are moving in a positive direction, things mutually and simultaneously develop. That is why the Yoga Sūtra uses this word aṅga. It tells us that the aṅgas must grow together.

Niyamas, like yamas, are attitudes and are not to be taken as actions or practices. The five niyamas are more intimate in the sense that they are attitudes we have towards ourselves. The first niyama is śauca, or cleanliness. There are two parts to this, external-internal. External śauca or cleanliness is simply keeping ourselves clean. Internal śauca has to do with cleanliness of the internal organs and mind. The practice of āsanas or prāṇāyāma could be an internal śauca.

The second niyama is saṃtoṣa, a feeling of contentment. When we act, we pin our hopes on certain anticipated consequences. We are often disappointed. In such moments we should not feel despair. We should accept it. That is contentment and it is a highly respected concept. There is a commentary on the Yoga Sūtra which says that contentment is greater than sixteen heavens combined. If there is contentment, we can always achieve spiritual happiness. Instead of despair when our actions don't yield desired results, we progress and learn from our actions. Saṃtoṣa has bearing on mental activities, such as study, on physical efforts and even on how we earn our living. Saṃtoṣa is about ourselves, what we have, and how we feel about what God has given us.

The next niyama is tapas, a word we have already discussed. Tapas means to keep the body fit. It is like heating the body to cleanse it. With tapas the idea is to bring out aśuddhi, "dirt" inside the body. Āsanas and prāṇāyāma are tapas, a means to keep oneself fit. Consideration of what we eat or how we eat is a form of tapas. If we are not hungry and we eat, we are doing the opposite of tapas. Posture, attention to food habits, breathing, are all tapas that help us to avoid the accumulation of "dirt" in our bodies. "Dirt" also means being overweight and short of breath. Tapas serves to make the body fit.

Svādhyāya is the fourth niyama. As we defined it earlier, sva means "self or pertaining to ourselves." Adhyāya means "study, inquiry, etc." Actually, adhyāya means to go near. Svādhyāya means to go near yourself, that is, the study of yourself. Any study, reflection, or contact that helps us understand more about ourselves is svādhyāya. We are encouraged to read ancient texts because our reaction to what we read will tell us something about ourselves. If we read the Rāmāyaṇa, the story might appeal to us and this tells us about ourselves. We cannot simply sit and reflect upon ourselves. We need some external reference such as the Bible, the Rāmāyaṇa or the Yoga Sūtra. Sometimes svādhyāya is taken to mean the repetition of mantras. If we have a guru who knows us very well, our strengths, weaknesses and interests, he might give us a mantra. When we repeat that mantra we come into "contact" with our guru; we look at his way of life, how he solves problems, etc., so that we receive guidance. The Yoga Sūtra says that the more we go into svādhyāya the more we are in contact with the laws of God, the teaching of the ṛiṣis (sages), etc. What we come in contact with depends upon the type of svādhyāya we do. If we read the Ramāyāṇa, we will know more about Rāma and his acts and teachings. If we chant the mantra our guru has given us, that guru will be our reference and rescue us. By rescue we mean that memories of him will guide us in our actions.

The last niyama has also been mentioned before. Īśvara-praṇidhāna means "to leave all our actions at the feet of the Lord." Since our actions often come from avidyā it is possible that they might go wrong. That is why contentment is so important. This attitude suggests that we have done our best, therefore we leave the fruits of our action in the hands of something higher than ourselves. In other words, we leave the rest to God. We will go into detail about Īśvara later.

Question: How do the kriyās relate to śauca?

Response: This is one concept not mentioned in the Yoga Sutrā. The word kriyā means action but in this context it is better understood as a purification process. An "outside" agency is used to clean the "inside." As an example, if our nostrils are stuffy, they can be cleared by pouring a very mild salt water solution through them. Suppose we have congestion resulting from smog. To clear our lungs we use a fast breathing technique. This concept is probably a part of śauca.

Question: I have seen tapas translated as austerity.

Response: If austerity means to fast just for the sake of fasting or to observe some strict and unaccustomed lifestyle for the sake of discipline, it is not tapas. As in the case of satya, any means of tapas we use must do us good. Simply to fast for twenty days without reason could cause us great difficulties. If by austerity we mean austerity with reason, it is tapas. Tapas must not make us suffer. This is very important.

The third aṅga is āsana. In the theory of āsana practice, you remember there are two aspects--sukha and sthira. We must be comfortable and at ease (sukha) and we must be steady and alert (sthira). We must be involved and at the same time attentive. Yoga suggests two ways to achieve these qualities in āsana. Locate certain knots or resistances in the body and by certain means release them. We achieve this progressively using the concepts of vinyāsa and counterpose. The means we use to release these knots must not adversely affect our bodies. We must plan carefully. If we force our bodies, the reaction will be negative and painful. Gradually the body will accept an āsana and we will be comfortable in it, able to breathe, able to feel the posture.

The second suggestion is to have a mental image of a perfect posture. An explanatory metaphor exists in Indian mythology, represented by Ananta, the king of the serpents. The concept of Ananta is that a cobra is carrying the universe on its head and at the same time is providing a bed for Lord Viṣṇu. The cobra must be relaxed to provide a comfortable bed for the Lord. That is the sukha concept. Yet the cobra cannot be dull and weak because it is carrying the universe. That is the sthira concept. These two qualities give us the idea of a perfect posture and how it should feel. To achieve this we must find the knots and the means to release them.

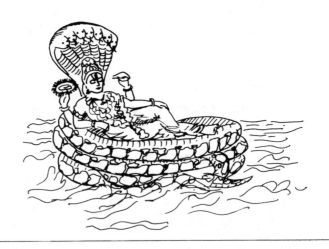

Ananta

Fig. 59

A very interesting thing is said about the effects of āsana. In life there are opposites, as Madras in May and

Hamilton in January. It is said that if we really know how to use āsanas we will be able to handle opposites. It does not mean that we can go bare-chested in cold weather or wear woolen clothing in the heat. However, because we know how the body behaves, we become sensitive, we know how to adapt. A test for āsana practice is our ability to adjust easily to extreme cold and heat. More practically, if we need to stand for a few minutes, we should be able to stand; if we need to sit for a few minutes, we should be able to sit. That is one advantage of doing āsanas. It helps us to get used to different things. When we practice prāṇāyāma, we need to be able to sit comfortably for some time. Āsanas help us to forget the body so we can pay more attention to breath in prāṇāyāma.

So far we have covered three of the eight aṅgas--yama, niyama and āsana. The next aṅga is prāṇāyāma and we will postpone a detailed discussion of it until later. Until then, a simple definition will suffice. The word has two parts, prāṇa and ayāma. Prāṇa means "breath." Ayāma means "to extend, to stretch." The practice most concerned with the breath is called prāṇāyāma.

IX

Practice

THE PRACTICAL ASPECTS OF PRĀṆĀYĀMA

Before I explain the practical aspects of prāṇāyāma, it is necessary to remove any unwarranted apprehensions about this practice. It is often asked if the practice of prāṇāyāma is dangerous. Be assured that just as we can do any exercise, such as āsana, so, too, we can do prāṇāyāma. In prāṇāyāma we simply breathe. As long as we observe how the body is responding to our breathing, we have nothing to worry about. Problems develop only when we insist upon holding the breath for a long time without paying attention to the reaction of our bodies. Some people think that long holding of the breath after inhalation and exhalation is a quick way to progress and they overdo it. In such cases problems can develop. As long as we follow our practice rules, to watch, to go gradually, etc., anybody can do prāṇāyāma.

It is not necessary that we sit in padmāsana or any other particular posture to do prāṇāyāma. However, it is important that we choose a posture we can stay in for a long time and get out of without feeling numb. Some people find kneeling very comfortable; others can sit in the lotus posture easily; and, in the beginning, it is even all right to sit in a chair. It is only important that the back be straight. There are times when we ask people to recline in a lounge chair to do breathing exercises. People with heart trouble need this. The important principle is that the body should not interfere with the breath. In prāṇāyāma we are dealing with the breath. In āsana we are concerned primarily with the body. While we use the breath for the body in āsana, in prāṇāyāma we accept the posture and forget the body. The only requirement is that we must be comfortable and keep our backs straight.

There are many types of prāṇāyāma based on different techniques and ratios. The easiest way to feel prāṇāyāma is just to observe the breath, feel how the breath goes in and out, observe the movement of the abdomen and chest. This is a basic type of prāṇāyāma.

The next type emphasizes inhalation. This is called pūraka prāṇāyāma. Pūraka means "to fill in." Pūraka prāṇāyāma is a long timed inhalation, a hold for one or two seconds, and then a free exhalation. A free exhalation is simply to wait for the body to expel the air.

Next is a very useful type of prāṇāyāma called recaka prāṇāyāma. Recaka means "exhalation." In recaka prāṇāyāma there is free inhalation, a hold for one or two seconds and a long timed exhalation. This type of prāṇāyāma is often used for relaxation. For someone who is very tense recaka prāṇāyāma is very useful. Through some special techniques it is possible to develop a lengthy exhalation.

Then there is kumbhaka prāṇāyāma. Kumbhaka means "to hold, to stop the breath." Here we hold the breath after inhalation or after exhalation or both. In this type of prāṇāyāma the attention is upon holding the breath. Inhalation and exhalation are free. As we noted before, for working in the chest area, but not including the heart, we use pūraka and kumbhaka after the inhalation, and for problems in the abdomen we use recaka and kumbhaka after the exhalation. For problems such as tension or anxiety we use only recaka prānāyāma. In certain cases of depression or dullness we use pūraka and kumbhaka after inhalation. If we want to calm ourselves, we use recaka and kumbhaka, and if we feel lethargic we use pūraka and kumbhaka after inhalation.

Another possibility in prāṇāyāma is that we can fix ratios between inhalation, holding the breath, exhalation, again holding the breath. There are many ratio possibilities that can be classified under two general headings. The first is called samavṛtti prāṇāyāma. Sama means "equal," vṛtti means "move." Samavṛtti prāṇāyāma is prāṇāyāma in which inhalation and exhalation are equal and if the breath is held, this too is equal to inhale or exhale. We often describe a breath, containing inhalation, holding the breath, exhalation, holding the breath, in numerical ratios expressed in seconds. For example:

Inhale	Hold after Inhale	Exhale	Hold after Exhale
10 seconds	10	10	10
10	10	10	0
10	0	10	10
10	0	10	0

This samavṛtti prāṇāyāma is very useful for people who use mantras in prāṇāyāma. They have a mantra that takes a certain amount of time. They can then repeat their mantra an equal number of times during inhalation, holding the breath, exhalation, and again holding the breath.

The other general type ratio in prāṇāyāma is called viṣamavṛtti. In this the breathing is not equal; therefore, there are quite a few possibilities. For example:

Inhale	Hold	Exhale	Hold
10	0	20	0
10	10	20	0
10	20	20	0
6	24	12	6

The last is a classic ratio of 1-4-2-1. This can be quite difficult.

There are different techniques for breathing. One of them is "throat inhalation, throat exhalation." By "throat," we mean the utilization of the same restriction in the throat that we described for use in āsanas. A variation of this is called anuloma ujjāyī prāṇāyāma. Ujjāyī means "that which clears the throat and masters the chest." We inhale through the throat and during exhalation we close one nostril completely and the other partially and exhale through the partly closed nostril. This helps to extend the breath. When using this nostril control, we do not use the throat restriction. Likewise, there is a technique

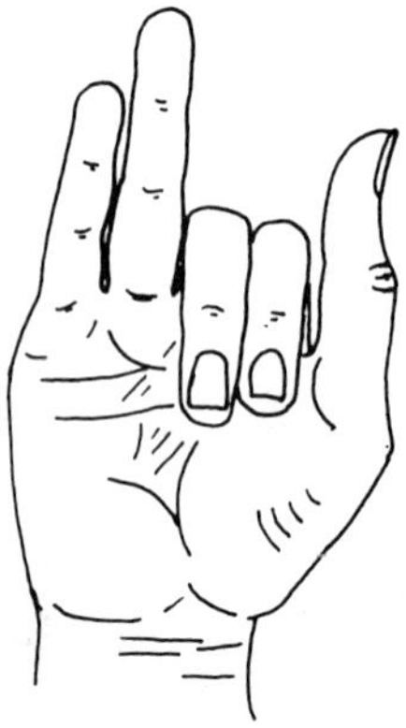

mṛigi mudrā

Fig. 60

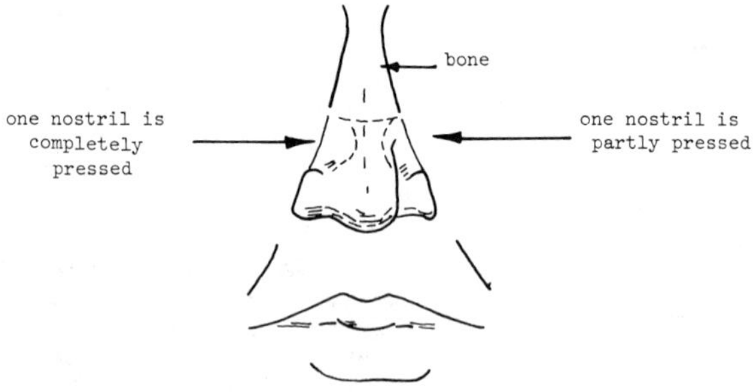

inhale, exhale through partly closed nostril

Fig. 61

called *viloma ujjāyī prāṇāyāma* in which nostril control is used for inhalation. Exhalation is with the restriction in the throat. This is a useful technique for those who wish to extend inhalation.

To extend both inhalation and exhalation there is a technique of alternate nostril breathing called *nāḍī śodhana prāṇāyāma*. *Nāḍī śodhana* means "that which clears the passages through which the breath goes." *Nāḍī* means "passage," *śodhana* means "purification." In this *prāṇāyāma* we inhale through the partly closed left nostril, exhale through the partly closed right, inhale through the partly closed right, exhale through the partly closed left, and so forth. The control of the nostrils is used by the hand position called *mṛgi mudrā*. (See Figure 60.)

To repeat, the idea of the partly closed nostril-breathing technique is to extend the length of breath, our inhalation and exhalation. Theoretically we can use any ratio for any of these techniques. In actual practice we do not do this. In *anuloma ujjāyī prāṇāyāma* we have limited control over the inhalation, so ratios with extended inhalations are impossible. In *nāḍī śodhana prāṇāyāma*, however, it is possible to do both *samavṛtti* and *viṣamavṛtti* types of ratios because both inhalation and exhalation are controlled at the nostril. A warning about alternate nostril breathing; if you have a problem with a nostril, say a blockage, you will not be able to use it. If you try to use force you will develop complications. To use nostril breathing we must be sure our nostrils are clear. If they are not clear, go back to throat breathing. We normally practice *ujjāyī* for a long time before introducing *nāḍī śodhana prāṇāyāma* in our practice. There are many more combinations and techniques.

Another useful breathing technique in *prāṇāyāma* involves the tongue. During inhalation we slightly turn up the two sides of the tongue and breathe through this passage. The technique is to curl the tongue like a tube and to inhale through it. As we inhale the air passes across the tongue which is usually moist. The air becomes cool and it refreshes the throat. To make sure that the tongue

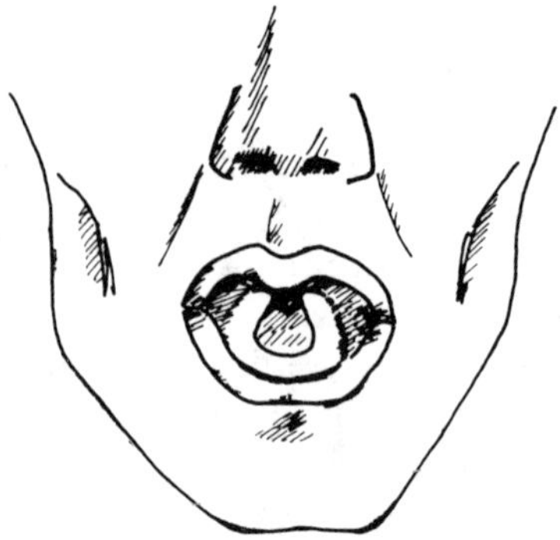

tongue position in śītalī

Fig. 62

remains moist, after inhalation and during exhalation, we roll the tongue backwards as far as possible against the roof of the mouth. This keeps the tongue wet so that the next breath will be as refreshing as the first. Exhalation can be done either through the throat or through alternate nostrils. This technique is called śītalī prāṇāyāma because śīta means "chill." It is impossible for some people to curl the tongue in this way. If this can't be done, we create the same effect of śītalī prāṇāyāma on inhalation by parting the lips and teeth slightly and placing the tongue gently back of the space between the teeth. This causes the air to pass over the tongue. Exhalation is through the throat or alternate nostrils.

There is also one type of breathing used for cleansing. If we have much phlegm or feel congestion, fast breathing is useful. Rather than extend the breath, we deliberately make it fast. To do this we use only abdominal (diaphragmatic) breathing; we do not use chest breathing. In this technique our breaths are short, fast, and forceful. We are using the lungs as a pump and this creates so much pressure in the expulsion of air that it forces out any "dirt" in the lungs. This very fast, powerful abdominal breathing is called kapālabhāti. Kapāla means "skull." Bhāti means "that which gives brightness." Kapālabhāti is the practice that removes heaviness in the head. For example, when we have sinus trouble, we may feel heavy around the eyes as if we are drowsy. Kapālabhāti might help to clear that area. There are modifications of this technique. If one nostril is blocked, we force the air in quickly through the clear nostril and out through the blocked one. This is called bhastrikā prāṇāyāma. Bhastrikā means "a bellows." It is called such because the abdominal movement during the breathing looks like a bellows. These two techniques vary greatly in different schools of yoga. The general principle is that we use the pressure of the air to clear the nostrils.

We must be very careful with these techniques. With this fast breathing we might feel dizzy. Therefore, when we do kapālabhāti we always follow it with slow breathing. Suppose we want to do one hundred fast breaths. It would be best to do about twenty-four fast breaths and then four to six slow breaths with long exhalations, then twenty-four fast breaths followed by four to six slow breaths with long exhalation, etc., ending with the slow breathing. There is no holding of the breath with this slow breathing because that would also cause hyperventilation.

Transition to the practice of prāṇāyāma should be made gradually and progressively. After āsanas we must rest a few minutes before prāṇāyāma because in prāṇāyāma the orientation is toward the breath, not the body. This intervening time not only gives the body a rest, it helps the mind make the transition. Without rest there will be tension because we will want to make a transition and the body will be unable to accept it. Therefore we must always rest.

How do we construct a ratio? Suppose we want to do a ratio of 10-20-20-0. We begin by investigating our inhalation and exhalation. We must first establish our inhalation and exhalation ratio before holding the breath can be introduced. Otherwise we will become tense during practice. First, we would try to do six breaths of 10-0-20-0. If we could not do this, it would be foolish to try a more complicated ratio. We would have to pick another ratio. However, if we could do 10-0-20-0 easily, our bodies would be ready. We would then introduce some holding of the breath, for example, 10-10-20-0. This might be satisfactory for four breaths but no more. On the fifth breath we might notice that our exhalation is getting shorter or our inhalation becomes unsteady. We would not proceed but go back one step and use 10-5-20-0. For this particular day 10-5-20-0 would be a good ratio to use and it could be repeated for about 12 breaths.

If we carefully fix a ratio for each day and investigate our capacity to do it, we will really understand and benefit from prāṇāyāma and never hurt ourselves doing it. As in āsanas, we move progressively investigating each breath before we attempt another. This is particularly important if we use a prāṇāyāma with a long kumbhaka. For example, if we want to do a ratio of 6-24-12-0, the following would be a good introductory progression:

Inhale	Hold	Exhale	Hold	Ratio
6	6	12	0	6-6-12-0
6	12	12	0	6-12-12-0
6	18	12	0	6-18-12-0
6	24	12	0	6-24-12-0

If we can do six breaths of the first ratio and six breaths of the second ratio, we can then try 6-18-12-0 for six breaths. If this is satisfactory we can go on to the next ratio 6-24-12-0. However, if this ratio is unsatisfactory, we must return to 6-18-12-0. At times we might be able to do higher holding ratios, at times not. It depends upon the condition of our bodies. If we have eaten much heavy food, our breathing will not be good the following day. If we have done the proper and the right amount of exercise, if the lungs are clear and the stomach is not full, our breathing will be good. Remember, we always progress gradually, mastering the first step before we go to the next.

There is one more thing to be said about prāṇāyāma with holding of the breath; that is, the concept of ascending and descending. Suppose we want to do an 8-8-8-8 ratio. We don't start with this but do the following:

Inhale	Hold	Exhale	Hold	No. of Breaths
8	0	8	0	6
8	8	8	0	6
8	8	8	8	6
8	0	8	0	6

First we try six breaths without holding the breath. If that is comfortable, we then try holding the breath after inhalation for six breaths. Then, if that is all right, we go on to the peak or longest ratio. We descend with 8-0-8-0. If we do postures, rest and immediately begin our prāṇāyāma with the higher ratio, we might not be able "to be with the breath." There will be tension. To avoid tension we begin with a simple ratio, gradually ascending to a peak and descending to a simple ratio. This principle in the practice of prāṇāyāma must be followed. It is important to do this descent since it is like a counterpose after the peak ratio. It takes only a short time and is worth doing. Gradually we can increase the number of breaths in the peak ratio.

Mental attitude is very important in the practice of prāṇāyāma. In prāṇāyāma we have no body movement to see; it involves mostly what we feel. The only thing dynamic in prāṇāyāma is the breath. Yet, we must have the same attitude of attention in prāṇāyāma as in āsana. To follow the movement of the breath we should feel inhalation from its beginning at the collar bone down to the diaphragm. Exhalation is the opposite, beginning with a contraction of the abdomen. This is the easiest way to concentrate upon the breath. While there are many other techniques, for now, we should simply follow the movement of the breath inside the body. Another beginning technique is to feel the breath only at the place where it enters or leaves the body. To focus on the breath at the nostril means that we must use the alternate nostril technique to make a sound. This sound is simply a vibration and is influenced by the flow of air. Here we try to keep the sound of the breath uniform. We can also follow the breath by the sound in the throat. These suggestions will keep us in touch with what we are doing, otherwise, our prāṇāyāma exercises will be mechanical. Even the ratio of inhalation and exhalation is not as important as our involvement with the breath. Timing is only an aid to being involved in the prāṇāyāma. The objective of giving different techniques and ratios in prāṇāyāma is to give us a variety of approaches by which we can follow the breath. When we follow the breath, the mind becomes more and more involved in that activity. This concept in prāṇāyāma prepares us for dhyāna, meaning, "the mind is ready to go in one direction."

Question: When you are using alternate nostril breathing, do you also use the throat restriction?

Response: No. The idea of using the nostrils is to regulate the breath at the nostrils, not the throat. If we practice carefully we will find that it is very difficult to get sound from both the nostril and the throat. The sound comes from a change in pressure. The air flows at a higher velocity because of the restriction of space in the nose or throat. If the change in pressure is in the throat, it cannot also be in the nostril. We could train ourselves to get the sound at both places, but the idea, however, is to regulate the breath either at the nostrils or in the throat.

Question: Can you relax the diaphragm during the period of holding the breath after inhalation or exhalation?

Response: If we are inhaling properly, there is no need to relax the diaphragm. If we are using the ribs to expand the lungs more than they can easily do, the diaphragm is sucked up too high. If after inhalation we feel a slight restriction in our throat, we have lifted the diaphragm too much and need to relax it. On exhalation, if we contract the abdomen too much the air rushes out too quickly and we cannot control its flow. Also, if we have completely exhaled and still we continue to contract or pull the abdomen inward, air flow during the subsequent inhale cannot be controlled. In fact, if we get a choking sound as we begin to inhale, we have contracted the abdomen too much. All of this can be felt in the throat.

Question: After exhalation should the diaphragm be relaxed?

Response: If we are contracting the abdomen too much, we must relax. This also applies if we are contracting the abdomen too much after inhalation.

Question: You said we could either follow the breath or concentrate on the sound at the place where it enters the body. Should we consistently use one of the techniques throughout a particular practice session or can we switch back and forth?

Response: It varies but before we discuss this, let me comment upon the number of breaths we take in a given session. It is said that if we are doing one practice session we should do at least twelve breaths. The number of twelve has been suggested because it is an Indian time-honored system of counting with the fingers. Since on each hand we have twelve finger segments, not counting the thumb, begin counting by placing the thumb on the lower segment of the index finger and proceed through twelve counts as follows:

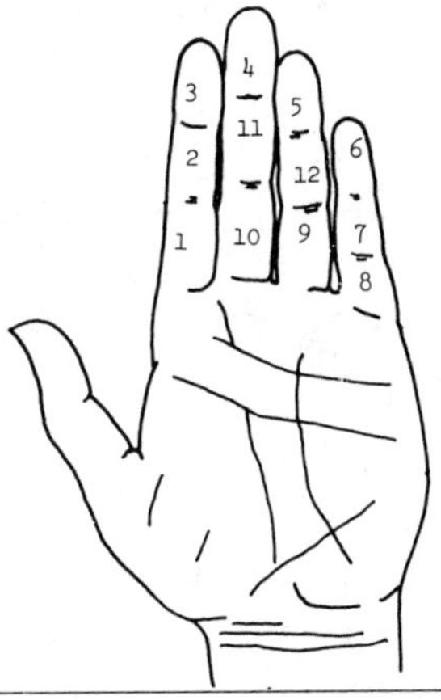

thumb starts at 1 and moves to 2, etc.

counting the number of breaths in prāṇāyāma using finger segments

Fig. 63

Now, about your question, I think it is better to stay with one technique of concentration; either by following the breath or by concentrating on the sound of the breath. It is much easier to discover something while concentrating on one technique rather than spreading our attention. If we do twelve breaths of one type and then twelve of another we might change our point of concentration because the different ratio will change our mental attitude. The area of concentration depends upon the ratio and type. If we do 8-0-16-8 for twelve breaths the point of our attention will be the abdomen. Whereas, if we do 6-24-12-0, the point of attention will be the chest; that is, keep attention on the area where maximum effect and effort takes place.

Question: Could you comment further on the technique of just following the natural movement of the breath?

Response: It is really difficult simply to follow the natural movement of the breath because once we focus upon the breath, it tends to behave differently. We tend to control or to interfere with its natural rate. It is "something" simply to follow the breath. The natural movement of the breath centers in the diaphragm. When we follow the natural movement of the breath we tend to do one of two things--either we will feel the movement and be involved in it, or we will feel it as a witness. As a witness we have nothing to do with the activity. We are like a man watching the flow of a river. If we are able to do this, it is almost a state of meditation. That is why it is sometimes suggested simply to watch the breath. Doing this is to still the mind. That is not easy but it is wonderful.

Question: I find it difficult to keep count while holding the breath.

Response: That is interesting. Holding the breath gives us a moment when there is nothing happening. A moment when it should be possible to count. In fact, the best time to introduce mantras is not during inhalation or exhalation but while holding the breath. It is said that a moment of holding the breath is a moment of dhyāna. Some mantras are very long. Since we do not have to concentrate on breathing while holding the breath, these longer mantras can be recited correctly. So I am surprised at your question. Perhaps you should try to use the finger counting method. With this you can do wonders. Merely place the thumb on a joint to note the breath and beat the thumb on the joint, one beat for each second, to count the length of the breaths. Perhaps this will help.

Question: Should we eventually be able to do prāṇāyāma without counting?

Response: Yes. What is prāṇāyāma but "to be with the breath"? This is very difficult and that is why we have so many techniques. Normally our bodies have their own rhythm and we are not conscious of our breathing. By counting we become consciously involved with the breath. Some people say prāṇāyāma is boring. They say that just to sit and do breathing exercises is quite ridiculous. There appears to be more challenge in postures; they produce a visible result in terms of form. Still, if we are completely involved in prāṇāyāma, who cares what the numbers might be? Number and type, ratios and other techniques are only a means, not a final goal. That goal is not to need any technique. If we can just be involved with the breath, an active witness to the breath, that is prāṇāyāma, the highest prāṇāyāma. But this is easier said than done.

Question: Will you say something more about holding the breath after exhalation?

Response: I did give you some idea of its use for problems in the abdominal area. I can add that holding after exhalation is usually more difficult than holding after inhalation. If you want to do a ratio of 10-10-10-10, I would suggest the following progression:

Inhale	Hold	Exhale	Hold
10	0	10	0
10	10	10	0
10	10	10	10

If you can do the first ratio for six or eight breaths, then try the next ratio. If neither inhalation nor exhalation is affected, then you can try 10-10-10-10. However, if you are more interested in holding the breath after exhalation, it might be better to do 10-0-10-10.

Question: Should ratios always be balanced in factors of one to two or could we do something like 6-0-9-0?

Response: In theory, yes; however, it is better to have a balanced relationship between the parts of the breath. It makes it easier to count.

One more advantage of holding the breath after exhalation is that it will help us make exhalation longer. If our ratio is 6-0-9-0 and we want to increase the nine to twelve, one of the easiest ways to do this is to introduce a progression like this:

Inhale	Hold	Exhale	Hold
6	0	9	0
6	0	9	6
6	0	12	0

Always be sure you can comfortably do at least six or eight breaths of a ratio before you move to the next progression.

Question: Are the more difficult prāṇāyāmas done only in simple postures? How would you integrate prāṇāyāma in a sequence of āsanas? You said that in prāṇāyāma the body should not get in the way of the breath, and that a simple comfortable posture is best. Is it best to do the difficult prāṇāyāmas as a separate practice after you have completed a practice of āsanas?

Response: Yes, exactly. We always finish our āsanas, rest a few minutes, and then sit in a comfortable posture and do prāṇāyāma. Suppose we want to do 5-0-10-0 for twelve breaths. That would take only about three minutes. For three minutes there might be several postures that are all right. Suppose we want to do

10-10-20-0 for twelve breaths. That would take us about eight minutes. In this case it is obviously better to go to a simple posture. The longer we want to do prāṇāyāma the simpler the posture must be.

Question: Is it necessary to prepare for prāṇāyāma in a difficult ratio the same way every day?

Response: While it really could be different every day, some preparation is always necessary. If we are aiming at a particular ratio and use āsanas intelligently our preparation could be relatively brief. For example, if we want to hold the breath after both inhalation and exhalation, we won't want to do a lot of strenuous postures.

Question: Do you always do prāṇāyāma after āsanas?

Response: If we are doing āsana practice, then it is better to do prāṇāyāma afterwards. Āsanas, unless they are too strenuous, help achieve good breathing. There are exceptions but generally we do first āsanas and then prāṇāyāma.

X

Theory

THE FOURTH AṄGA--PRĀṆĀYĀMA

Before we proceed, are there any questions about our last discussion of yama, niyama and āsana?

Question: Would you go over the definition of ananta? I have often seen it translated as "infinity."

Response: In the Yoga Sūtra two means are suggested to bring the qualities of steadiness (sthira) and ease (sukha) to our practice of āsana. The first is to locate and release certain knots or resistances in the body using the principle of progression. Āsana is a position of the body in which we are at ease and at the same time active and firm. The second means is to have a particular mental attitude toward the concept of ananta. The word anta means "end." An-anta means "no end." When doing an āsana we should have an image of a perfect pose. While ananta is often defined as infinity, how can we relate this idea to the definition of āsana as being firm and at ease? Fortunately, we have been given the image of Ananta, the king serpent, who provides a comfortable bed for Lord Viṣṇu and at the same time a protective umbrella on which he supports the whole universe. (See Figure 59.) Infinity does not make sense in the context in which we are working. Ananta can also mean breath and what is suggested here is the use of breath in establishing an āsana.

It is a mistaken concept that certain āsanas are only postures for meditation. If we look at the commentary of Vyāsa, we see that the postures he elucidates are so complicated that we can't be in dhyāna. We can feel these different postures and we can't stay in them. Two of these are uṣṭrāsana and krauñcāsana. These are very difficult postures in which to remain. It is very clear that the postures given are not only for meditation, but are of value in enabling us to stand for a long time, to sit and to adjust

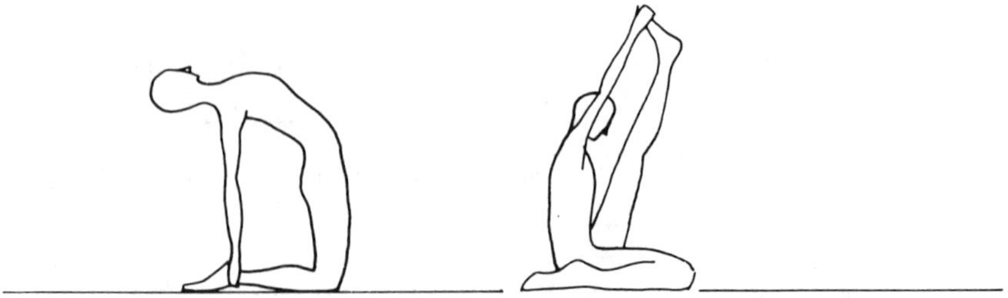

Fig. 64

to different circumstances.

Let us continue with prāṇāyāma, the fourth aṅga. Prāṇāyāma is the suspension of the normal movement of the breath. We focus our attention upon the breath. Whether it is to control the breath or simply to observe it, our first objective is to be conscious of the breath. The Yoga Sūtra says that prāṇāyāma is when we become conscious of the breath. Next we determine how to continue to be conscious of it, that is, how to "remain present with the breath." One suggestion is to control or regulate inhalation and exhalation. It is also suggested we choose a place in the body where we can feel or hear the breath. This we call deśa. These aspects of prāṇāyāma we have already discussed.

The word prāṇāyāma has two parts, prāṇa and ayāma. Ayāma means "to stretch or to draw," and this is the active part of prāṇāyāma already described. Prāṇa means "that which is constantly present everywhere." The breath is constantly coming from somewhere within the middle of us. As long as it is there we are not dead. In the following diagram we have an aura of prāṇa both within and around us. It is almost as if this prāṇa is radiating out

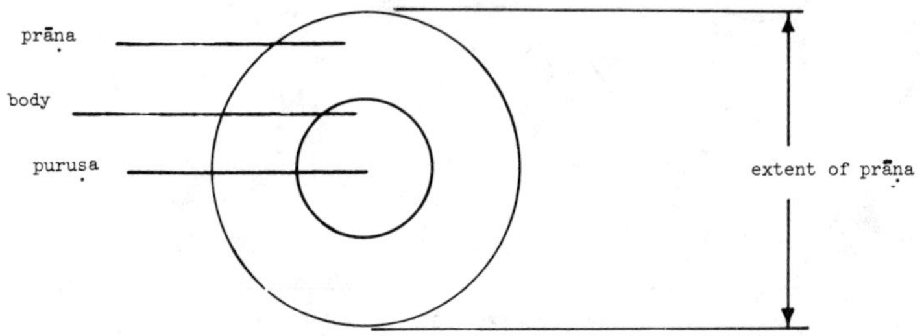

the extent of prāṇa increases if a person is excited, confused, or sick

Fig. 65a

from the center all through the body and a little beyond. Different sources explain prāṇa as a friend to puruṣa. Prāṇa is simply the expression of puruṣa in all parts of the body and beyond. This prāṇa has an intimate relationship to the mind because the puruṣa sees only through the mind. Thus prāṇa, mind and breath are interrelated. Whatever happens in the mind influences the breath. That is why the pulse rate increases and breathing becomes faster when we are excited, and why breathing becomes very deep and the pulse is quiet when we are relaxed. The mind/breath relationship is an evident fact. In prāṇāyāma we use the breath to do something with the mind so that the prāṇa increases its intensity. Tradition tells us that an unsteady person, one who is confused, has more prāṇa beyond the body than within it. The measure of prāṇa beyond the body is more when we are not at ease and therefore, the prāṇa within the

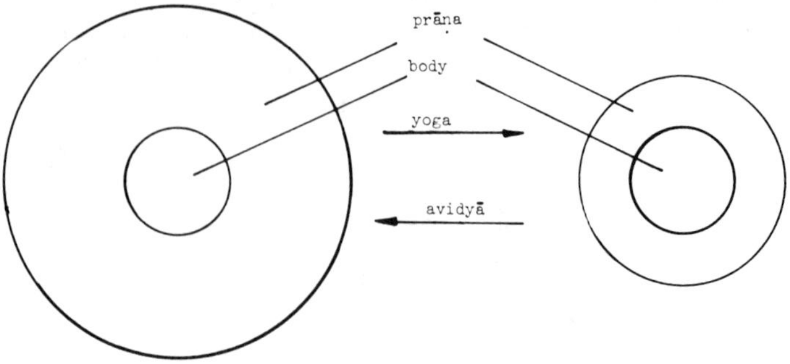

yoga practice draws prāṇa closer to the body

Fig. 65b

body decreases in quality. The measure of prāṇa beyond the body is less when we are quiet. What we are trying to do in the practice of prāṇāyāma is to confine more and more prāṇa within our bodies. When prāṇa is not able to enter our bodies, it is because something is there that should not be. The Yoga Sūtra uses the word kleśa, "defilement" but let us call it "dirt." To review, prāṇa is the expression of puruṣa and it is within the body and beyond. The more a person is content or at ease, the more prāṇa is within. The more a person is disturbed, the more prāṇa is scattered. In prāṇāyāma we hope to bring the measure of prāṇa outside the body down to zero. In fact, one of the definitions of the word yogi is "one whose prāṇa is within the body." If the prāṇa is not within the body, one is not a yogi. This is the symbolic representation of the word prāṇa and its relation to us. To influence the prāṇa we have to influence the mind. In prāṇāyāma this is achieved by means of the breath. In life, our actions often disturb the mind and increase the measure of prāṇa outside the body. We reverse this process by the daily practice of prāṇāyāma. The Yoga Sūtra says that as we practice prāṇāyāma, more and more of the covering of the mind, avidyā, is removed and there is clarity. The mind becomes fit for dhyāna. When disturbance of the mind is reduced, the prāṇa is more within the body. The idea is to bring prāṇa within ourselves so that we are our own masters.

Question: Does prāṇa go out with the breath as you exhale or does it stay within you?

Response: An answer to this will be somewhat speculative because there is no direct proof. We can only sense this by our state of mind. If we are consciously linking breath to mind it is as if we are linking prāṇa. We use this link in yoga practice. When we inhale it is as if the

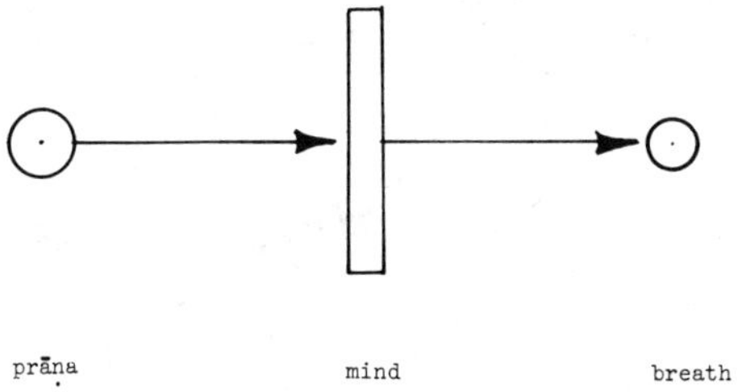

breath linked to prāṇa through the mind

Fig. 66

prāṇa goes in. When we exhale, it is as if whatever prāṇa cannot stay in the body goes out.

There are five prāṇas, vital forces of the body. They have different names depending upon their association with functions in the body: prāṇa-vāyu, udāna-vāyu, vyāna-vāyu, apāna-vāyu, and samāna-vāyu. We will concern ourselves with the two basic pranas, prāṇa-vāyu and apāna-vāyu. Prāṇa-vāyu centers in the chest. Apāna-vāyu is responsible for excretion. Apāna also represents the center where body waste collects. Sometimes that which enters the body is called prāṇa and that which leaves is called apāna. There is a lot of confusion over the word apāna. Let us understand it simply as meaning prāṇa that is located and accumulated where it should not be.

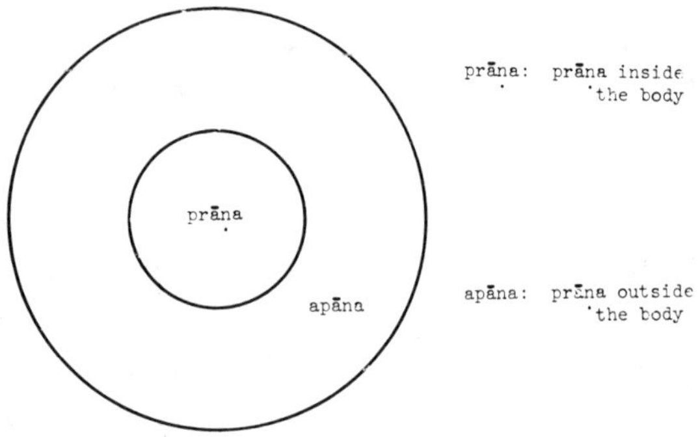

location of prāṇa and apāna

Fig. 67

Question: Does the same thing occur when we control breathing in āsana?

Response: Yes, to some extent. However, in āsana attention is divided between the breath and body movement. In āsana we use the breath as the medium of movement to affect the body. Since our attention is divided between body and breath the effect upon prāṇa will not be as much as in prāṇāyāma.

Question: Is the point to rid oneself of some prāṇa or to leave all the prāṇa in?

Response? The point is to have the maximum prāṇa inside the body. This will become clearer when we explain more fully the difference between prāṇa and apāna. One definition says that conscious inhalation is prāṇa and conscious exhalation is apāna. In that context we said that apāna is that which goes out of the body.

Let us continue in our consideration of prāṇa. On inhalation the idea is prāṇa that is outside the body is brought in towards the apāna. During inhalation prāṇa meets apāna. During exhalation the apāna that is within the body moves towards prāṇa. The more impurity a person has in the body, the more apāna increases. We de-

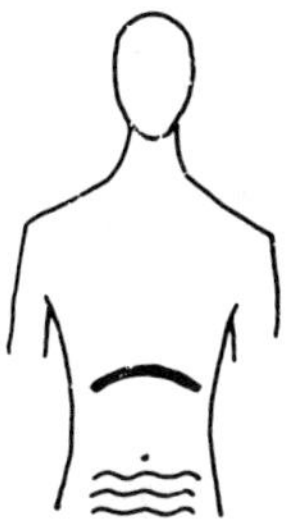

apāna: defilement in the body

the location of apāna

Fig. 68

crease the apāna so that we can bring more prāṇa into the body. Anything we do to reduce the dross in the body is a forward step. The concept behind a ratio such as 10-0-20-0 is to provide a longer time during exhalation to rid the body of wastes. Apāna, "defilement, dirt," accumulates in life due to factors both within and beyond our control. Our action in yoga is to reduce this. A person who has shortness of breath, who cannot hold the breath, or make longer exhalations is considered to have more apāna. A person with good, comfortable breath control is thought to have less apāna. The more apāna we have, the more problems we have in all areas of the body.

Prāṇāyāma is a movement of prāṇa towards apāna and a movement of apāna towards prāṇa. Holding the breath after inhalation brings the prāṇa towards the apāna and holds it there. Holding the breath after exhalation does the reverse. Let us next consider what is happening in this movement of prāṇa, apāna.

One of the concepts in yoga is that we have a fire inside our bodies, and it is located somewhere between prāṇa and apāna. The seat of this fire is near the navel, but the flame itself shifts. On inhalation there is a downward movement of the breath. This downward movement

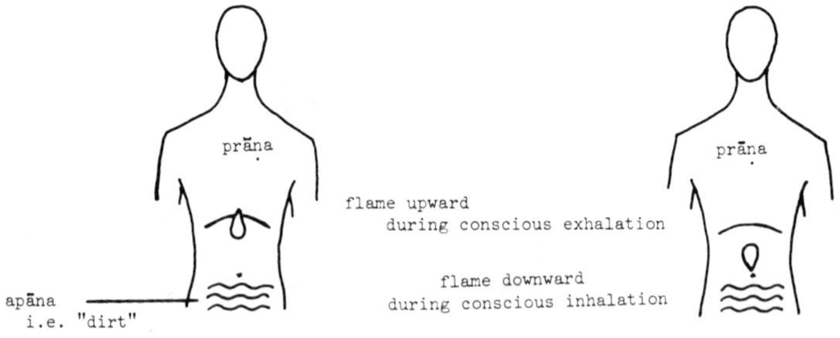

the concept of the fire

Fig. 69

of breath creates a draft, as in a flue, which draws the flame downward. It is this flame that burns the "dirt" from the body. During exhalation the draft works the other way, it brings the "burnt dirt" out. The job of burning the "dirt" takes place during the inhalation and holding the breath after inhalation. When exhaling, the burnt apāna or "dirt" goes towards prāṇa and then on out of the body. This is the job of prāṇāyāma.

Question: In light of what you said, wouldn't a long inhalation to burn the dirt be more desirable than a longer exhalation?

Response: Importance is given to exhalation to allow for more time to remove the "dirt." It is not enough to burn the "dirt," we have to expel it. Longer exhalation is suggested to give every chance for the "dirt" to go out. On the next inhalation we can bring the flame back to the "dirt." It is important that all the "dirt" burned leaves the body.

Question: I understand that holding the breath after inhalation theoretically gives more time for the flame to burn the "dirt." What is the reason for holding the breath after exhalation?

Response: It is not enough that we bring the flame towards the "dirt." It is also necessary to bring the "dirt" towards the flame. That is why when we exhale and hold the breath after exhalation we use certain bandhas, physical body "locks" or contractions. Very gradually we develop the lower abdominal muscles so that we can lift the lower abdomen, the area of apāna, towards the navel and hold it there during the entire prāṇāyāma. This technique is called mūla bandha. After exhaling we bring the "dirt" towards the flame so that on the next inhalation, the effect of the fire is increased. Every part of the prāṇāyāma works together to remove apāna and bring prāṇa into the body. The moment there is no "dirt" the prāṇa goes into its proper place. Nobody can control the prāṇa, it has its own movement. We create a condition in which the prāṇa returns. There is a very good simile given in the fourth chapter of the Yoga Sūtra. If a farmer's fields are terraced and he wants the water to flow down he simply breaks the upper dam. In prāṇāyāma we simply remove the "dirt" and the prāṇa goes in. It is beyond our conscious effort to move the prāṇa. What is within our conscious effort is the breath, so we use the breath to make this movement possible.

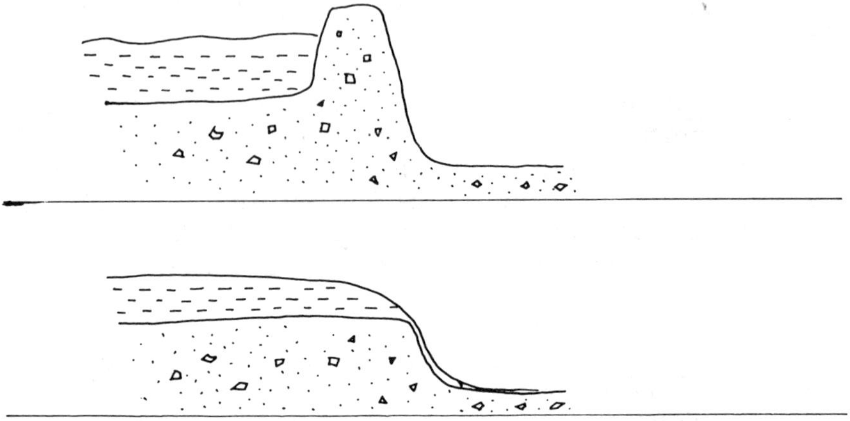

farmer cuts the bund for letting water into the field

Fig. 70

This same principle applies to inverted postures. Inverted postures bring the flame towards apāna. If we do prāṇāyāma in the inverted postures its effect is increased. That is why inverted postures are given so much importance.

Question: Are apāna and "dirt" the same?

Response: Apāna refers to the area of the lower abdomen and all activity there. It means that part of the prāṇa which is in charge of evacuation. When a person is heavy we say he has too much apāna. Of course we need a minimum of apāna which is a part of prāṇa itself. There are other prāṇas elsewhere. For example, one type of

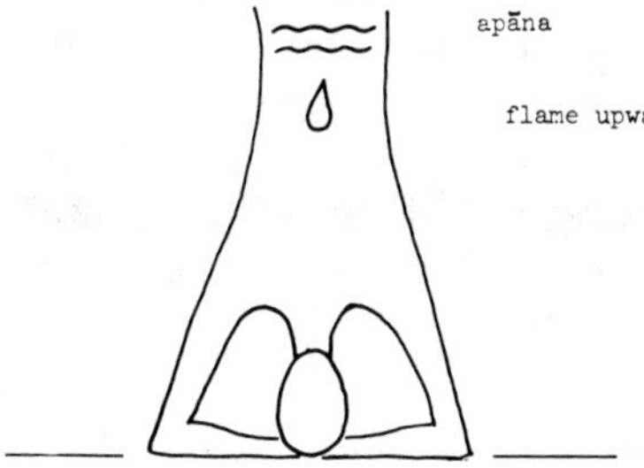

the concept of the fire in inverted postures

Fig. 71

prāṇa called udāna-vāyu centers at the throat. This prāṇa is responsible for speech. If we don't have udāna-vāyu in harmony, our speech is impaired. So all types of prāṇa are required but they must be in balance. If a person has dross in the lower abdomen he spends too much energy in this region. He has too much apāna and so needs to correct this imbalance. The idea is to reduce the apāna to the minimum, an efficient minimum.

Question: What is this fire in the body?

Response: It is the whole mechanism in the body responsible for producing heat. More than anything else it relates to the process of making the food we eat easier to assimilate. Some say that the fire is in the stomach. I would say it involves the entire portion under the diaphragm and above the navel. This fire is that part of the human mechanism that is responsible for "cooking" and producing heat. When we eat we sweat because our temperature rises during digestion.

Question: Did you say that we cannot directly affect the prāṇa by a conscious effort?

Response: Since we describe the prāṇa as an expression of puruṣa, we have no conscious means to effect it. We must work through the breath and mind. We can only make conditions proper for the prāṇa to enter.

Question: I was thinking about something such as an ulcer. In that case is the fire too strong? Can we decrease the fire in prāṇāyāma?

Response: We can control the fire by modulating the breath. A ratio of 20-0-20-0 will produce a greater fire than one of 6-0-12-0. If we make inhalation shorter, the fire is less. If we inhale longer, the fire increases. If we use the ratio 6-24-12-0, the fire also increases. There are some people who always feel heat in the body. For them we suggest the śītalī prāṇāyāma mentioned earlier. Never use long holding of the breath after inhalation. By making inhalation short and exhalation long we reduce heat.

The technical term for this fire is sūrya which means "that which is always hot."

Question: Does the fire burn only upon inhalation?

Response: The fire is always there. Conscious inhalation increases the fire and it brings it towards the bottom of the torso. If we do that and hold the breath for some time the fire can work on the "dirt" and give us the possibility of removing the "dirt" on exhalation.

Question: You said that prāṇa is the expression of the puruṣa. Would the prāṇa be in its place inside the body if there were no interference from the mind?

Response: That is exactly the idea!

XI

Theory

ANTARAṄGA SĀDHANA--AN INTRODUCTION TO THE LAST FOUR AṄGAS

You have had enough time to give some thought to the material we covered in the previous lectures. Do you have any questions?

Question: In the last lecture you explained that a yogi is one for whom all the prāṇa is inside the body. Why is this desirable?

Response: The ideal is to have the prāṇa inside the body. For this to occur, there must be nothing to prevent it from being inside, meaning that the negative, the "dirt," is no longer there.

Question: How does the yogi know that the prāṇa is inside his body?

Response: He will know if it is outside by the many symptoms which indicate that something is wrong. If nothing is wrong, that means the prāṇa is inside the body. The Yoga Sūtra mentions certain things that indicate something is wrong within us. It might be a feeling of duḥkha, we don't know what is wrong, but we know something is wrong. It might be a disinclination to act. Other times the breath might be short or the whole body trembles. When there is no disturbance of mind or shortness of breath or other symptoms, the prāṇa is inside the body. If on the other hand we have one problem or another at some time or other, then prāṇa is outside the body. The concept of prāṇa inside or outside the body can be understood symbolically to represent a state of mind. In the state of mind where the mind is like clear glass, there is nothing to corrupt the body, there is no "dirt." On the other hand, if there is always a hesitation to act because there is a possibility of wrong action, then there is "dirt" in the body. This "dirt" is present not only at the physical level, but even more so at the mental level. Anything that is "dirt" in the body must be understood as having originated from avidyā. To say that a yogi is a man who has everything in him is a symbolic way of saying that he is the master of himself. We cannot say simply that because the breath is related to the mind, and therefore to the prāṇa, that when we inhale, the prāṇa literally goes inside the body. It does not happen this way. Prāṇa enters the body the moment there is a positive change in the state of mind. Of course, the state of mind will not change on every inhalation or exhalation. It changes over a period of time. When we do prāṇāyāma and it has an effect upon the mind, it means that prāṇa has already entered the body.

Question: The point is clear that avidyā does not always manifest itself. When avidyā is not manifest there can be moments of clarity though the seeds of avidyā might still be there. How can we distinguish between a true moment of clarity and a moment of self-deception?

Response: What is a moment of self-deception? In self-deception there is a division within ourselves, unless we are such experts at self-deception that this division does not occur. That is why the yamas and niyamas are very important. We can know about self-deception, however, through external relationships. If we are proper and respectful in our attitude towards people, this will tell us whether there is self-deception or not. I might think that I am the greatest yogi, but through what people think of me, how they relate to me and how I relate to them, I know exactly whether I am or not. That is why it is important to live in this world with people, to see what response there is between us. Otherwise, we could easily deceive ourselves.

Question: I can see how these yamas and niyamas through something like a conscious effort of the will can bring about a reduction of avidyā and its effects. Is that the method through which we finally suppress confusion, yielding to certain temptations, desire, hate, etc.?

Response: We have to consider what is cause and what is effect. Very often cause and effect are confused. We might follow a certain course of conduct in life, expecting to attain a specific goal. Very often it will not happen. But, in the process of life, through a personal evolution, things might happen, things we did not expect to happen. You see, yamas and niyamas might be effects as well as causes. At one time we might tell a hundred lies and still feel happy inside. Later we might feel a reluctance to tell a lie. This is the progress of yama. We cannot look ahead with certainty to see what will happen. We can only see, for example, what has happened from 1972 until today. That might be a hint of what will happen tomorrow.

Question: Do we just constantly watch these things arise and then try to stop them?

Response: We must first watch. As we know, the first prajñā is to say, "Look here, something is happening, let me be careful." We don't just take to the highway and go to a place. We have to be constantly watching.

Question: Isn't that easier for someone living in a place like Chapel House than someone working and living with a family in the everyday world?

Response: Both might help. A friend of mine who came to India thought being in the Himalayas for two or three years would help him. He managed to find a good place and stayed there for three years, quite alone. He had some books, and did what is called sādhana, intense practice. I don't know what kind of sādhana it was. He then came to me to check about some postures and to study the Yoga Sūtra. Upon his arrival in Madras, he said that he felt a lot of things had happened to him. He seemed very delighted. He used complex terms like sabīja samādhi to explain his evolution in the Himalayas and this pleased me. He found a small place in the compound of the Theosophical Society in Madras, a very quiet place with no disturbances, lots of trees, and an excellent library, etc. After two days he came to me and said he had changed his mind and was going to find a big place to live. Knowing him for five years I was a bit surprised. I asked him why he wanted a big house. He said, "You know, I met a girl. My whole life is changed now." While I am not condemning this change, I want to point out that what he thought he was, he was not.

So, Chapel House can help, but the real test of Chapel House would be in Madras. And the real test for someone from Madras would be to see how they feel in Chapel House. I'm sure some people cannot stay here for more than a day. Someone not sure of himself can't live in Madras long either. So change helps. We have to see both the fire and the water to know how we will react. We have to test ourselves in different situations. That is why yama is important. It involves our relations to and with different people in different circumstances. Then we can know what we are.

Question: Is changing environment important to yoga?

Response: Yes, some changes are very important. The mind gets so used to things that our actions are really habits, saṃskāras. We will never know our real nature unless we go to another environment. That is why we must test ourselves by going to the other side. If a man cannot get along with people, how can he say he has understood himself? Once in Europe a friend came to see me. He thought his whole life had changed after yoga. He gave up meat, smoking, hashish, all those things. He led a very strict life. He came to me one morning and saw me drinking a cup of tea. He was shocked. He couldn't stand the idea of his teacher taking tea. He said, "How can you take tea?" I asked what had happened to him and why he was so worried about the tea. I told him, "You seem to be more affected by this tea than I am." We must be able to live in the midst of people to test ourselves, to see whether we understand ourselves. This is, I think, the true test. This is what I mean by having the prāṇa inside the body. When this is the case, a person is not affected by the whims and opinions of others.

Question: I understand how we can restrain ourselves from acting on a desire we recognize as bad. At this point, should we be concerned with this restraint rather than trying to understand how to reach a point where the desire wouldn't arise in the first place? I get upset about the fact that the desire arose. And then I worry about getting so upset. It all works in a sort of circle.

Response: It is a question of seeing whether what we think is a problem is really a problem. Consider what is meant when we say "something bothers me." To see whether something is really a problem, it is often helpful to shift environments and see from a new perspective how the same situation might appear. For example, you have an occasion to tell a lie. At the moment, it seems convenient, so you feel like lying. You then feel bothered, thinking "How can I tell a lie? It is better either to keep my mouth shut or to tell the truth!" How do you know? We can talk to someone about it abstractly and see their reaction. There might be certain "white lies" that avoid serious social interactions. Similarly, a lie might avoid spending too much of our lives pursuing each individual situation. Or the lie might be of no consequence. So we discuss it with somebody else, or we change the environment and look at the situation afresh. We find an occasion in which we can reflect again. That is why the *Yoga Sūtra* says, if something bothers us, think of the opposite. We might find that what we think bothers us is not really the source of our worry. We find a situation that provides us with a different setting; we read a book, we talk to a trustworthy friend, we go to a cinema. At that moment when we are not clear about what to do, we should never act.

Question: At the moment of doubt we should never act?

Response: If there is time, do not act. If there is no time, find some time, make some time. At the moment of doubt it is best to stop. I'm sure quite a few actions could be stopped.

Question: It seems that at the moment of doubt often

it is impossible to stop, particularly when we are responsible for other people. In real life situations, the time of most doubt, our tension is often because we cannot stop. If we could stop, the strain would probably not be so severe. So when there is doubt, do we look to something else, do we confront it, do we ignore it?

Response: It is not always enough that we find a situation where we can reflect. Somehow we must be able to look at the same problem from a higher point. This change of vantage points is a form of evolution. Through yoga we are a little better today than yesterday and therefore we can look at the same problem in a different way. Otherwise by reflecting from the opposite direction or talking to someone we try to cope with problems but we don't improve ourselves by going beyond these problems. What is important in yoga is that there must be growth. We must evolve so that what was doubt need no longer be doubt. For example, for me to change my career from engineering to yoga, in 1964, was a major decision with weighty problems. I had talked to many people, and the problems still remained. Then one day it was no longer a problem. I looked for the problem from a different, higher point and it was no longer there. It is also true that sometimes the more we try to clarify something the more it becomes a problem. What is important is that we try to be a little better. If we are a little better, doubts tend to vanish. All the aspects of yoga aim at making us a little better so that we have fewer doubts about our actions. We must strive and wait to be better. We will not be confronted with as many problems as before. Sometimes we might stop striving, but over a period of time we will have to improve. Whatever helps us to improve, we must do.

Question: A few lectures back you were talking about changing the state of mind. You said that this happens when something makes an impression upon us and drives us in a particular direction. What enables us to stop or change direction? Suppose I have a desire and at the same time feel that I would like to get rid of it. Does puruṣa act or, if not, what enables me to act?

Response: In your example two elements are present, a desire and a hesitation. Suppose there is desire to have some fun, why should we hesitate? Desire is not necessarily a problem. We should not intellectualize normal life into great problems. If somebody invites me for a cup of coffee and because coffee does not agree with me, it becomes a problem, something is wrong. It is a lesser problem simply to say yes than to explain why I believe coffee is bad. Similarly, certain desires need not be problems but we make problems out of them intellectually. Suppose we desire marriage. That is something we have time to think about and we should not be in a hurry. Classify the desires into two kinds: desires that are incidental and of no consequence, in which we can simply act this way or that, and desires that we must stop to think carefully about. Experience will tell us what really matters and what does not matter. In things that matter, we generally have time. In that time we can reflect and we can change. We can always improve ourselves so that the problems resulting from desire become smaller.

Does puruṣa act in this? The action of puruṣa, which is to see, is always there. Puruṣa acts but only through the mind. When we are talking our puruṣa is involved in our talking. Whether or not the action will be regrettable depends upon the state of mind; if the mind is colored, the action is colored, if the mind is clear, the action is clear. Our aim in yoga is to have a clear mind so that the effective action of puruṣa is perfect.

Question: Is puruṣa's only action seeing or can puruṣa motivate action?

Response: Puruṣa is the energy for action. Motivation is also an action and therefore puruṣa is involved in it. Puruṣa is involved in everything because puruṣa is the energy to act. But since puruṣa always acts through the mind all our actions are not perfect. The action depends on the quality of the mind. We are trying to change the quality of mind, so that the quality of action gets better and better.

Question: Is puruṣa contained in anything?

Response: We say that puruṣa is in the body. To some extent the body is the container of the puruṣa, but not in the sense that the body is holding the puruṣa. Whether there is a living body or not, there is puruṣa. It is not like a box in which puruṣa is put. So it is not confined tightly within the body.

We can now proceed with antaraṅga sādhana, an aspect of yoga in which there is no form of practice. We have discussed the first four aṅgas, yama and niyama as attitudes and āsana and prāṇāyāma as two limbs we can practice. The remaining four aṅgas are called antaraṅga sādhana, meaning "certain things we really cannot practice, rather they just happen." All we can do is to prepare ourselves for them to happen. Antara means "within," that aspect of the body that is inside us, the mind and the senses.

YOGA

Bahiraṅga (can practice)		Antaraṅga Sādhana (cannot practice)
Attitudes	Practice	pratyāhāra
Yama	Āsana	dhāraṇā
Niyama	Prāṇāyāma	dhyāna
		samādhi

Let us discuss pratyāhāra, the fifth aṅga that involves the senses, a very difficult subject! The word āhāra means "food." Pratyāhāra means "withdrawing from that on which we are feeding." This refers to the senses. When the senses refrain from "feeding on" their objects, that is pratyāhāra. If there is a beautiful sunset, our eyes are drawn to look at it. That is the normal way the senses function. It is possible, when we are completely absorbed in something, that even though the beautiful sunset is there we won't be seeing it because our absorption is in something else. Normally, by habit, the senses tell the mind, "Look here," "Smell this," etc. The senses register an object and the mind relates to that object. In pratyāhāra we cut this relationship so the senses withdraw, the senses don't function. The objects for the senses--for the eye, form; for the ears, sound; for the nose, smell, etc.--are before the senses but they don't function. The senses are not allowed to be influenced by their objects. This is called pratyāhāra. For example, if we are completely absorbed in the breath in prāṇāyāma, automatically there is pratyāhāra. The mind is so involved with the breath that the link between mind, senses and their objects other than the breath is severed. Pratyāhāra is that state in which the senses do not relate themselves to objects. It is not a state of sleep. The senses are capable of action but do not act because they are uninfluenced by their objects. They are withdrawn.

For example, you ask questions and I try to clarify the subject in light of those questions. The more I become involved, the more I don't even recognize where I am. I become absorbed in our interaction, which itself is a state of pratyāhāra. Even though my eyes are open, I am so involved in what I am saying that my senses don't function. Pratyāhāra does not mean we look at an object and say, "We are not going to look at that object." The moment we focus upon the object we are going to look at it, unless we close our eyes. We create a condition in which the mind is somehow, somewhere so involved that the senses don't respond to the object.

Question: We talked earlier about a spirit of detachment. Does pratyāhāra involve this detachment?

Response: If I see something and say, "I don't want it," that is not pratyāhāra. In this, one part of the mind says, "Come, let's have it," and the other part says, "No."

Reply: I am referring to action and acting completely.

Response: How can it be pratyāhāra? In action we might have to use our senses. I am involved in talking to you and I have to use my mouth, my ears, etc. The notion of detachment means although we act, we are not always thinking about what we are going to get as a consequence of that action. That is vairāgya, detachment towards the fruits of action. Pratyāhāra is related to the senses. The senses are there. In a state of meditation pratyāhāra is automatic because the mind is completely with the object of meditation. In pratyāhāra the senses do not function in the usual sense due to the mind's involvement in something else. The importance of this is that the senses often become very sharp. But in our normal life situation due to conditioning, they become our masters. They make us crave to eat, etc. In pratyāhāra it is the opposite. If we need to eat, we eat, but not just because of a craving. We are really trying to put the senses in their proper position, not to cut them from action.

Question: Is pratyāhāra a means to control a physical discomfort by focusing our attention on something else?

Response: This is a possible effect of pratyāhāra. Suppose we are sitting in padmāsana and we are completely absorbed in what is God or Om. We don't even know we are in padmāsana. When we come back to ordinary awareness we have to massage our legs, etc. Something was happening in our legs but we were not aware of that because our interest was somewhere else. In that way it is possible to mask pain. To shift the mind towards another object of the senses in order to intentionally forget the pain is difficult because the senses are always working collectively. Pratyāhāra is a state that happens spontaneously.

The sixth aṅga is dhāraṇā and it too is a part of antaraṅga sādhana. Dhāraṇā comes from the root dhṛ, "to hold." There is a traditional example given to explain dhāraṇā. Suppose there is a tank of water with channels extending from each side. If the channels are of the same depth, the water will flow equally in them all. If we dig one of the channels deeper, more water will flow in that one. That is an example of dhāraṇā. Dhāraṇā is when we create a condition so that the mind, going in a hundred different directions, is directed towards one point. We create a condition by inquiry, etc., in which this is intensified. We encourage a particular action of the mind and as this action becomes more intense, the other movements

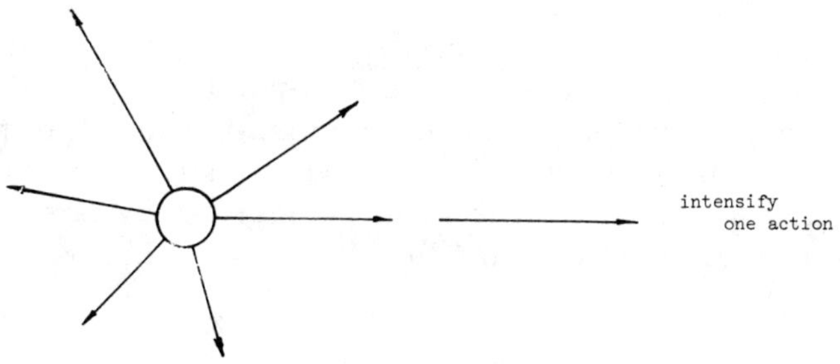

a distracted mind with movement in all directions

dhāraṇā

Fig. 72

gradually subside. That is dhāraṇā. It is the state of mind where the mind orients itself towards one point and nowhere else. It could be anything, but only one thing. Dhāraṇā is a step leading towards dhyāna. In dhāraṇā the mind is moving in one direction, nothing else has happened. In dhyāna, when we become involved with a particular thing and we begin to investigate it, there is a link between myself and this thing; that is, there is a perceptual and continuous communication between my mind and the object. If there is this communication, it is called dhyāna. Dhāraṇā must happen before dhyāna. The mind must be directed towards a particular goal before there can be communication. When the mind becomes involved in one particular object and nothing else, and communication takes place, it is dhyāna. Dhāraṇā is the contact. Dhyāna is the communication. Further, when we become so involved in an object that our mind completely merges with it, that is called samādhi. In samādhi we are almost absent, we become one with that object. We lose our personal identity in the sense of name, job, family, bank account, etc. In that moment all those things are gone. There is no mental gap between us and the object. They merge. That is samādhi.

To review: In dhāraṇā we establish contact with the object; the mind is oriented towards a single object. In dhyāna, there is a growing communication; the mind is fully attentive to the object. When that communication becomes so deep that the mind is completely absorbed with the object, that is samādhi.

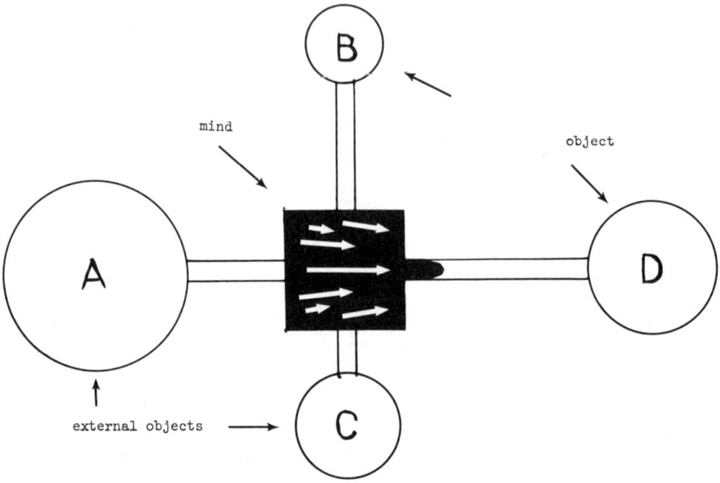

dhāraṇā: the mind is oriented towards a single object

Fig. 73a

Remember, we don't practice dhyāna. In the Yoga Sūtra the whole subject of dhāraṇā, dhyāna, samādhi is not explained in the chapter that describes practice. It has been placed in the third chapter where the effects of yoga are discussed. In fact I can't sit here and say I am going to do dhāraṇā. Perhaps I can create conditions that encourage something like dhāraṇā. Āsana and prāṇāyāma can, according to the Yoga Sūtra, create a condition where the mind is fit for dhāraṇā. We need a particular condition of mind to do these things. We can't be returning

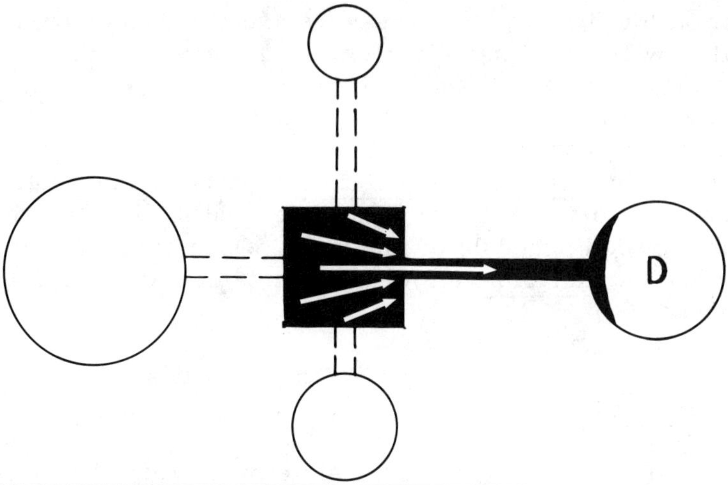

dhyāna: the mind fully attentive to the object

Fig. 73b

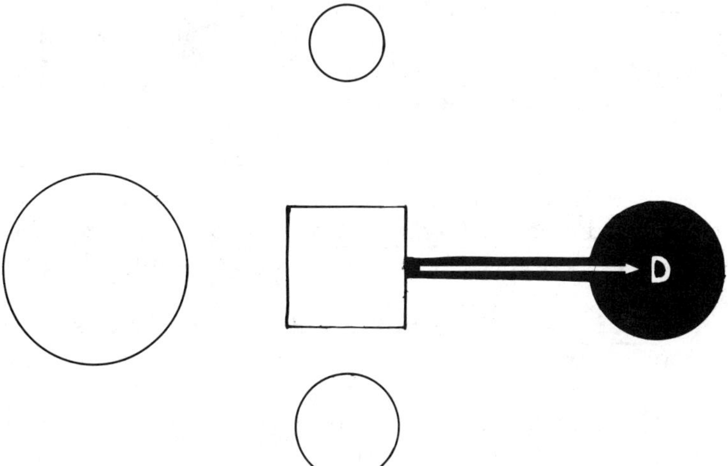

samādhi: the mind completely absorbed with the object

Fig. 73c

from a lot of shopping and say we are going to do meditation. Little by little we have to allow the hundreds of things going on in the mind to subside. If they are too powerful dhāraṇā cannot happen. And if we try to do dhāraṇā while various things are happening in the mind there will be conflict. That is why āsana and prāṇāyāma have been suggested because they affect the mental activity and slightly reduce that crowded schedule of the mind. Once dhāraṇā happens, dhyāna and samādhi can follow. Any other questions please?

Question: What is the relation between pratyāhāra and dhāraṇā?

Response: It is in the state of dhāraṇā that pratyāhāra occurs. The word pratyāhāra is used to explain what happens to the senses in a state of dhāraṇā. We can't be thinking of a hundred things and say, we are going to do pratyāhāra. Pratyāhāra is a result of a state of dhāraṇā, dhyāna, samādhi. It is put before dhāraṇā in the Yoga Sūtra, not because it occurs first but because it deals with the senses rather than the mind and is therefore a little more external than dhāraṇā. To say, "I am now going to do āsana, then I am going to do a half hour of pratyāhāra and then I am going to do dhāraṇā" does not reflect a correct process.

Question: Do we have to be sitting down in one place to do dhāraṇā, dhyāna, samādhi or is it possible to have that when looking at a sunset or something like that?

Response: Yes, in fact, it is helpful to use external objects, particularly in the beginning. That is why in all the temples we have statues, or, as in this chapel, a cross. It is to facilitate the beginner getting a feeling of dhāraṇā, but it is only a first step. Whether we sit or stand does not matter. We may be walking and still not feel the locomotion. There are certain schools in India that teach us to walk and meditate. If something like walking disturbs our dhāraṇā, our dhāraṇā is not very strong. But in the beginning it is always best to start with the easiest thing, a comfortable seated posture, and an object that is pleasant--something we like. Suppose we do not believe in Śiva and I say you must meditate on Śiva. There will be conflict. We must start with something that suits us. It is stressed in yoga that we have to start from where we are and with what we like. Finally the object does not matter. However, it is important that it does not bring conflict and prevent us from focusing in one direction. We suggest a certain object according to a person's temperament and belief. We must use such conditions that help us orient ourselves in one direction. If someone says, "I feel like walking and meditating," I don't see why not.

Question: What would be the difference between pratyāhāra in the sense that we are oblivious to what our senses are sending to the mind and another situation where we register it but choose not to respond? Say someone was involved in playing music and his senses register that somebody was waiting to talk to him. He could first finish his music and then say, "Yes, you wanted to speak with me?" Is that pratyāhāra or would pratyāhāra be that he didn't even know someone was waiting to talk?

Response: It should not be mistaken that in the state of dhāraṇā, dhyāna, samādhi the senses are dead. For example, we have some beautiful Sanskrit poems composed by some sages at the moment of samādhi. They sing. When we sing we use our senses, but in the case of the sages they use their senses for what? Just towards serving the mind. The senses don't distract the mind. It is not that the senses are dead. They only act in relation to the direction of the mind and not against that direction. These actions of the senses perpetuate the state of dhyāna. Is this clear? Suppose we are describing a beautiful image of God. We have to see the toes, the ankles, etc. That means we are seeing but our seeing is only for this context. If we see the feet and start thinking of them as stone and then about the geological context from which the stone was taken, or the particular kind of stone, the mind is distracted. If we see the feet and recognize them as the feet of the image and that they are like a lotus, then the senses are working in tune with the mind. Please don't have the impression that the senses are dead. In pratyāhāra they do function but just to serve the mind. Pratyāhāra is when the senses serve the mind in the state of dhāraṇā, dhyāna, and samādhi.

Question: Is it true that in the state of pratyāhāra there is perception? Is it just that the objects are immediately perceived without mediation, that there is no discursive thinking about it? Do we perceive but without mediated thinking?

Response: It depends. For example, there can be thinking involved in the example I gave of the image of God which is a part of dhyāna. Thinking is present but only in relation to the object and nothing else. Only the memory of this object is functioning. The pratyāhāra in this case allows no distraction by the senses because we are so involved in the object of meditation. The senses respond only towards this goal. If I am talking to you about the Yoga Sūtra and I smell nice food and I start thinking about the food, it is not pratyāhāra. But even if the smell is there, I continue to explain and my senses don't care, I am in a state of pratyāhāra. In dhyāna there is a medium for communication which could be thinking. In samādhi there is not even this thinking. There is a sort of thinking because there is understanding, but it is very minor. We can go deeper and deeper into this word samādhi. There are many states of samādhi--with ego, without ego, etc.--but I don't think we need to cover all of that. In dhyāna there is thinking. In samādhi the mind does not have to think because it is clear, it has understood as it is.

Question: I'm not sure of the distinction between dhāraṇā and dhyāna.

Response: Take for example how I begin any class here. I have been thinking and planning but I don't know exactly how I will proceed. So we begin and I ask if you have any questions about what we discussed last time. That is the beginning of dhāraṇā because I have not started communication, I am just orienting myself to talk about yoga. Dhāraṇā is only preparation and orientation. As I get more and more into the subject, dhyāna comes. In dhāraṇā I am more susceptible to distraction than in dhyāna. That is the difference.

Question: Let's say you were a student trying to write a paper and you have an idea. As you sit down and begin to orient yourself to that idea you are in dhāraṇā. When you really get involved in the effort to understand so that you can write, do you move into dhyāna?

Response: Of course.

Question: What would samādhi be in relation to this example?

Response: Suppose you are writing an essay and you get stuck in the middle. You don't know how to proceed. You must stop for a while and go somewhere for a change. But as you are doing this you suddenly get a flash--"I've got it!" From this you work backwards. You don't get the whole essay in your mind. You "got it," that is all. Then you come back and elaborate. Of course, this is far-fetched and a poor example, but it might be helpful.

Question: In dhyāna is there still a consciousness that I am thinking about this idea but in samādhi, all of a sudden it just comes?

Response: Yes, the gap is much less. In samādhi, the understanding is so close that we don't have to think as we do in dhyāna. The first chapter of the Yoga Sūtra explains how samādhi happens. First we reason, maybe it is like this or maybe it is like that. This is what we call vitarka and it uses much logic. Then vitarka stops because we can't go on back and forth. So we reflect. That is called vicāra, we think a little coolly. As this reflection is refined, asmitā samādhi occurs. Asmitā here means two things become one; the feeling "I am with it." Then we understand. At that moment we feel a state of blissful happiness. That is ānanda. We feel finally that we have understood what we wanted to understand. Actually, ānanda precedes asmitā in the Sūtras but they are similar. Ānanda is the expression of the experience of asmitā samādhi. Here asmitā refers to the merging of the mind with the object of meditation. This is the process of samādhi. First there is oscillation of the mind. Then superficial logic is reduced. The process becomes inward, deep and subtle. Then the reflection is very refined, a point comes where we know we have understood. There is no hesitation. The effect at that moment is the state of ānanda.

XII

Practice

CHOOSING A RATIO AND THE PROPER TECHNIQUE FOR PRĀṆĀYĀMA

Let us continue our discussion about the practice of prāṇāyāma.

Now, a very important aspect of the practice of prāṇāyāma is how to establish the right ratio for individual practice. We can't go on doing the same ratio. We might need something new to maintain our attention to practice or to suit a particular need. If the ratio is too easy, our prāṇāyāma will become mechanical. If it is too complicated or difficult, there will be resistance or conflict.

The choice of a proper ratio involves two things--what can be done and what should be done. What can be done involves a given person's capacity to inhale, hold the breath, exhale, and hold the breath. What should be done involves our direction of movement, our aim, our need. We have to accept where we are and move towards where we should go. This movement from a point where we are to a point we want to reach will always be present in yoga.

What can be done can be easily established if we observe our breath in āsana. If we observe how the breath fluctuates, how the body responds through the breath in certain postures, we will get an idea of the limits of our breath. Let us take, for example, three postures--a bending forward, a bending backward, and a posture in which the throat is restricted, such as the shoulderstand. Suppose I ask a person to try 10-0-10-0 in each of these postures. In the bending forward posture he can do 10 seconds of both inhalation and exhalation. In the bending backward posture he can't do either inhalation or exhalation for 10 seconds. In the shoulderstand, the exhalation is all right but the inhalation is short. We can see that this person has difficulty in prolonging inhalation. If we fix a ratio of

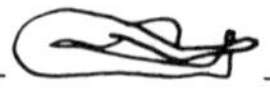	10 inhale 10 exhale	possible
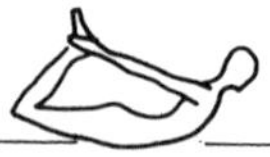	10 inhale 10 exhale	not possible
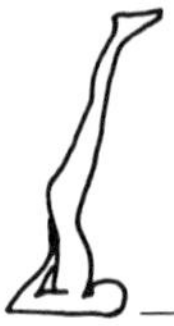	10 inhale 10 exhale	inhalation becomes short exhalation possible

remarks:

1. inhalation good bending forward
2. inhalation difficult bending backward
3. inhalation difficult in inverted posture, exhalation is alright

conclusion: probably has difficulty extending inhalation

Fig. 74

equal inhalation and exhalation and watch the breath over a period of time in certain postures, say for eight to twelve breaths, we can learn a good deal about the breath. In this example, the person probably could do a longer exhalation in prāṇāyāma, but might have difficulty doing a long inhalation. Such a person can perhaps use a ratio of one to two. I'll try to elaborate. If the person can do the desired length of exhalation while bending forward, he probably has nothing to obstruct the contraction of his diaphragm and abdomen and can execute the exhalation easily. Also he is able to make the exhalation in the inverted posture. In the shoulderstand the stomach and organs of the abdomen rest on the diaphragm. Normally, in such an inverted position it is difficult to exhale slowly because the weight on the diaphragm tends to make the air rush out. The movement of the air is like a piston. If a person, in spite of this, can control exhalation in this position, he will find exhalation easier than inhalation. An understanding of this is important, because it will guide us in the long run in planning our prāṇāyāma. Āsanas can tell us much about the body, including how the breath behaves.

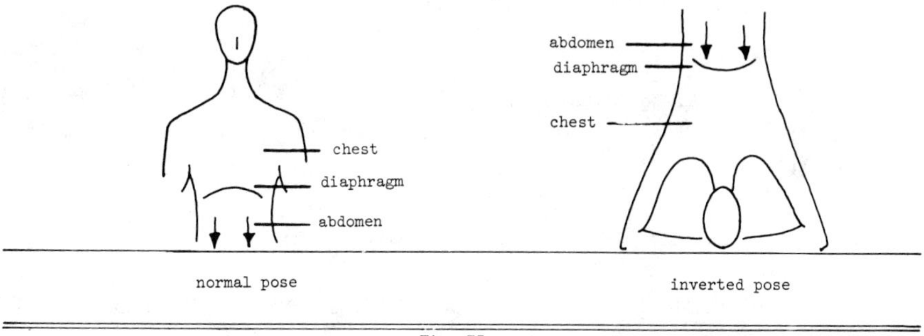

Fig. 75

<u>Question</u>: If we continue using <u>āsana</u> like that over a long period of time, wouldn't we eventually need to change our ratio?

<u>Response</u>: That is exactly what should be done. We find out what we can do and also what we cannot do. The person in our example can exhale but has a problem with inhalation. Obviously we will try to concentrate on extending the inhalation unless there are other related problems.

<u>Question</u>: Should we work on the breath in <u>āsana</u> using <u>prāṇāyāma</u> techniques?

<u>Response</u>: Why not? When we start doing postures, we are very attentive towards the breath. Earlier today I asked some of you to plan a program in which you would use not more than 120 breaths. (See Appendix.) This program included the headstand. The total number of breaths was all right but each breath was not. There was no union of breath and movement. You focused on the whole program that was planned rather than <u>each breath</u>. That is

why sometimes we have to invite our attention back to the breath. How can we do this? One way is to fix the duration of the inhalation and exhalation. It can be useful to fix the breath in basic postures such as the headstand or the shoulderstand. It is not always helpful to do it in the more complicated or dynamic postures.

Let us take another example using the same ratio, 10-0-10-0, and the same postures. In the bending forward posture and the shoulderstand the inhalation and exhalation are all right. The difficulty is with inhalation in the bending backward posture. The exhalation in this posture is all right. What does this mean? Any ideas?

Comment: It might be that the stomach is being stretched so much in the bending backward posture and the inhalation is difficult.

Response: You say it is because of the posture that inhalation is difficult and so it is not necessarily an indication of the breath. A good observation. Any others?

Comment: I would have thought inhalation would be more difficult in the other postures because of the contraction in bending forward and the throat restriction in the shoulderstand.

Response: So it would seem, but it has been observed this way. This is not easy to understand, but sometimes it happens. Sometimes the body can fool us. If we doubt such reactions we can find out by introducing something else into the postures. In this case, I would ask the person to hold five seconds after exhalation. That is, 10-0-10-5. Then observe. Sometimes people are so comfortable in postures, it is almost as if they are lying flat. To ensure that we know the problem, we introduce holding the breath after exhalation. Then the true quality of the breath is revealed. We might find that in this example, the exhalation becomes shorter and the inhalation will continue to get worse. Then we know that this person probably has a problem with exhalation. So even holding the breath can give an indication of what can be done and therefore, what should be done. Very often people who are supple have problems with the breath. It is not always an advantage to have a supple body. If we have that problem, we have to introduce holding the breath to find out what happens to the breath. Depending upon this, we can know our assets and liabilities. We are just touching this broad subject briefly to make us aware that as we observe the breath in postures it will help us to know how to do prāṇāyāma. At the same time it will help to bring our attention to āsanas. It is very important to be attentive to what we are doing. This is not always easy and, therefore, to introduce something like this can be helpful. When we investigate its effect, there is discovery. This investigation of the breath in āsana helps us to have a feeling of discovery and thus new interest and attention in what we are doing.

Question: Is it the inhalation or exhalation that is generally more difficult in bending backward?

Response: There is no definite rule because there are so many factors involved. It depends on weight, stiffness, the particular posture, etc. There are people who are very slim. They can hardly inhale while bending backward because their chests are so tight. That is why we should not use a complicated posture to investigate the breath.

Having determined what we can do, we want to establish a direction of movement based upon this information. Suppose a person can do a long inhalation and a short exhalation and we want to make the inhalation equal to the exhalation. For example, a person can do 15-0-10-0, and we want him to do 15-0-15-0. The first step for anyone, and this is very important, is to make the exhalation longer than or at least equal to the inhalation. There are many ways it can be done. Can anybody suggest what means to adopt so that this person can do 15-0-15-0?

Comment: Use alternate nostril exhalation to extend the breath.

Response: That is one answer. Come on, share

your knowledge.

Comment: Introduce holding the breath after inhalation?

Response: No, that is not part of the problem. However, holding the breath after exhalation would be useful.

Comment: I would suggest beginning with 10-0-10-0, and gradually working up to 15-0-15-0.

Response: How? Can you mention some figures?

Reply: Start with 10-0-10-0. Then try 12-0-12-0. And then try 15-0-15-0.

Response: Anything else?

Comment: How about using some āsana to get better control of the abdomen and chest muscles?

Response: Using āsanas is a good idea, that also works. Any other suggestions?

Comment: What about trying to regulate the exhalation by exhaling, holding a bit, exhaling, holding a bit and so on?

Response: Some of you may not be familiar with this. We have not mentioned it because it is too complicated for beginners. In this technique, called viloma krama prāṇāyāma, we take a complete inhalation and then break the exhalation. For example, exhale five seconds, hold five, exhale five, hold five, exhale five, hold five, and then inhale. I wonder if a person who can hardly exhale ten seconds would find this technique helpful, or even possible. It would not solve our model problem. Are there any other ideas?

Comment: Could we use kapālabhāti to strengthen the abdominal muscles?

Response: The problem need not be in the abdominal muscles. Even if it is, I'm not sure kapālabhāti will strengthen the muscles. It might even make them flabby. If you lie flat and lift the legs and breathe you can strengthen those muscles. I don't think kapālabhāti will do that, since in this activity the exhalation and inhalation is so short and quick. I also doubt it will help make the exhalation longer.

Comment: How about making the inhalation shorter, for example 5-0-10-0?

Response: What would be next?

Reply: Then we would build the ratio up in this proportion.

Response: I understand but let me give you my idea. There are good points in what some of you have said. We can find some postures that will make the exhalation longer, such as bending forward āsanas. Here is my approach.

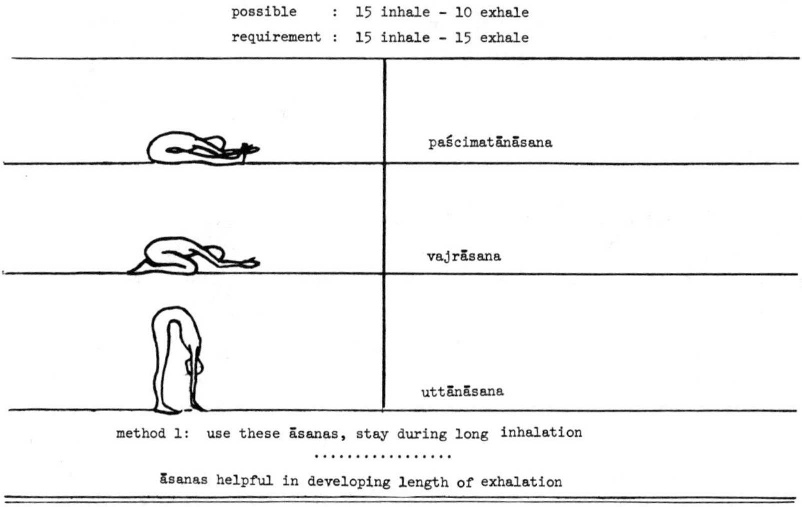

Fig. 76

The person is doing 15-0-10-0. Because the total length of the breath is twenty-five seconds he will also be able to do 10-5-10-0. This of course does not solve the problem. Next we introduce holding the breath after exhalation-- 10-5-10-5. This means exhalation plus holding the breath is fifteen. We now have a balance. After a week of this he can then try 12-0-12-0. If that is not possible through the throat, he can use nostril control to help.

Can do:	15-0-10-0
Should do:	15-0-15-0
First do:	10-5-10-5
After some days:	12-0-12-0
Then:	12-3-12-3
	12-6-12-3
	15-0-15-0

So a solution to what we should do might be simply to change the type of prāṇāyāma. If that is not enough, some special āsanas will help. The next thing is to introduce a little holding of the breath after inhalation and then gradually after exhalation. Then we can increase the exhalation. These are some of the means we can adopt. Such problems are solved through a combination of answers, not just one. Are there any questions about this?

Question: Can you review the first two suggestions again?

Response: The first possibility is to change the type of prāṇāyāma. There are many types. Lengthening inhalation or exhalation might be impossible using only the throat restriction. Then controlling the breath by the nostrils may help. If the problem is in strengthening and training the body, certain āsanas can be used. These are ways in which we can always keep some interest in the practice of prāṇāyāma. If we do the same thing every day, the practice will become mechanical. It is often good to change our practice. Also, over a period of time starting points and, therefore, goals will be different. If we respect these changes we will be able to adapt the prāṇāyāma according to the new situations.

There are certain exceptions. Some people need to do a particular type of breathing regularly. If we find that we are able to do 8-0-12-0, we might think the goal would be to do 12-0-12-0. However, there are cases where it is desirable to keep exhalation longer than inhalation. Thus the goal might be 8-0-16-0. There are people who become giddy, dizzy, or have a headache if inhalation is too long. In such cases or in cases where people want prāṇāyāma to be very relaxing, a short inhalation and long exhalation is better. So, our goals are not always to strive for what we cannot do. We then strive for what we should do. We must study the effects of various prāṇāyāma on ourselves and with this fix our ratios. We should be aware of another important point. There are people who find it easy to do 5-20-10-0 but what they really should be doing is 10-0-20-0. Even though they can hold the breath twenty seconds after inhalation, they cannot make their exhalation twenty seconds. They should practice the following progression:

Inhale	Hold	Exhale
6	0	12
8	0	16
10	0	20

These changes call for a gradual process and that can only happen over a period of time. At times we should do even less than what we are capable of doing. That is, 10-0-20-0 is only thirty seconds while 5-20-10-0 is thirty-five seconds. So remember, what should be done is what is helpful for us, not simply to do longer and longer sequences of breathing. The goal must be logically fixed. It is not like running a race.

Having briefly explained how to fix ratios in prāṇāyāma and how to use different types of prāṇāyāma, are there any questions about this before we turn to another subject?

Question: If our inhalation is shorter than our exhalation, does that mean we need to build up our chest?

Response: That is partly the case. We usually find that unless there are other problems, exhalation is longer than inhalation. I once had a flute player who could not extend the inhalation but she could exhale so well because of her training on the flute. In such a case, we must draw attention to the chest.

Question: Was her lengthy exhalation a matter of controlling the diaphragm?

Response: Yes, she was using the diaphragm extremely well on exhalation and then taking quick inhalations. Because of her practice with the flute she had to inhale quickly. The same thing happens with singers. They must use their ribs a little more. This means they must make the exhalations less so that the inhalation can be longer. In this case I would suggest the following progression:

Inhale	Hold	Exhale
3	3	9
3	6	9
6	0	6
6	6	6

This will, over a period of time, make a longer inhalation possible.

Question: What actually are we working on, the chest or the diaphragm?

Response: It can be both; however, it is mostly a matter of overall training. To attain a breathing sequence that is very long, training is necessary. There are people who can use the diaphragm very well but they don't have the training to make inhalation longer. Sometimes, of course, the chest doesn't expand or the stomach doesn't contract. With the flute player it was simply a matter of training. Are there any questions about fixing ratios?

Question: Are there guidelines that we can use to establish our goals? Should we be able to have a long inhalation or exhalation when we want it? Should we be able to hold the breath at the proper place?

Response: Yes. This flexibility is necessary, since the human existence is such that things change. At one time we might feel like doing a long inhalation and at another time we might feel like holding the breath. The aim in yoga is to train ourselves so that we can modify inhalation or exhalation and hold the breath to meet a demand. That is why we develop different ratios. If these things can be done, and if we need a particular ratio, it is in our pocket. However, we must be aware of immediate considerations. For example, if we are beginning students of yoga having done some postures and we would now like to do breathing, we do not set arbitrary goals. We do not say in one month we will hold the breath after inhalation, in two months we will hold the breath after exhalation. We must see what really suits us so that we become more and more interested in our practice. Gradually we can build up the time of holding the breath after inhalation or exhalation. This might have nothing to do with our immediate requirements. First, we see how the body responds to the breath so that we can follow the breath. If we can feel the breath and follow its movement, we will feel good after our prāṇāyāma. A feeling of well-being is not just having flexible joints, it is much more. Then we train so that any type of prāṇāyāma is possible. Both considerations must be there.

There are some other minor aspects of prāṇāyāma I would like to discuss very briefly before I turn to the concept of bandhas. We have already mentioned that in prāṇāyāma we must have a good posture, that we must select a type of prāṇāyāma, and that we must have a certain mental attitude, one of attention. We have noted that we can sense the sound of the breath or feel the breath as it moves through the body and that this helps focus attention. Something else that might help attention is a special form of gazing, that is, holding the eyeballs in a steady position but with the eyes closed. We use the eyes so often that it is not easy to keep them steady. Whether we are seeing, or hearing, smelling, or tasting, we somehow involve the eyes, thus the eyes are often overused. Closing the eyelids is a very important aspect of prāṇāyāma. We bring the eyes into a position as if we are looking at our abdomen, navel, tip of the nose, or between the eyebrows. Sometimes to bring an image to the eyes we envision certain things such as the full moon, the rising sun, or the reading of a mantra. In the beginning it is easier to do this technique of gazing during retention of the breath, forgetting about the position of the eyes during inhalation or exhalation. Internal gazing is not natural. Normally the eyes are always moving, even when closed. The attempt in any type of gazing is to hold the eyes at a fixed point. In a way, we are cutting off certain functions of the senses. The effect is to rest the senses.

Question: In the beginning, should we gaze only while holding our breath?

Response: Yes. That is the first step. If we start gazing while inhaling and exhaling as well as while holding the breath we might develop headaches because gazing is not a normal practice. In the beginning gaze only when holding the breath. It is easier, because there is no activity.

Question: How should we develop gazing?

Response: In the beginning we can gaze at the center of movement. On the inhalation we shift our gaze, our eyeball position, towards the solar plexus. We gaze there during holding. When we exhale we move the eyeballs downward towards the navel. A step beyond this would be to gaze at a fixed point regardless of whether inhaling or exhaling throughout the entire prāṇāyāma. First, we begin by gazing just during holding. Then we try it while inhaling and holding the breath. After a few months, we can gaze throughout the entire prāṇāyāma.

Another practice that helps our attention during prāṇāyāma is the positioning of our hands and fingers. These positions are called hasta mudrā. Hasta means "hand." The word mudrā has many meanings. Let us understand it as simply a symbol. We see these hand positions in paintings and sculptures of the Buddha. There are many possible hand positions. One called dhyāna mudrā is when we rest one hand in the other. Another is cin-mudrā. In it the thumb and index finger of the left hand join to form a circle and the right hand is used to modulate the breath at the nostrils. If our mind wavers during prāṇāyāma, our fingers will most likely separate. As far as possible the

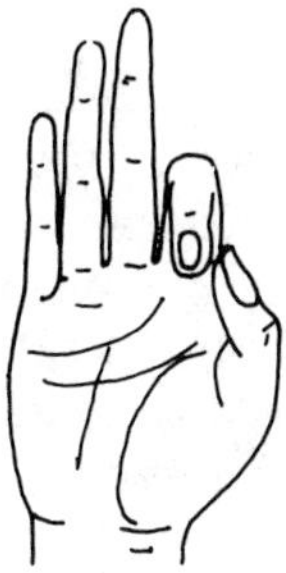

cin-mudrā

Fig. 77

whole body is used during prāṇāyāma so that we are sure we are with the breath. There are other ideas about mudrā. Some people say if we change the mudrā, we change the effect of the prāṇāyāma. We don't have time to go into all of these details. Just know that hand positions are one more way to tell us how far we were with the breath. If we fix a particular mudrā and after doing prāṇāyāma open our eyes and notice that our hands or fingers have changed positions, it means our attention was broken. This is a sort of check.

Question: Can't we become distracted by worrying about our hand positions?

Response: Yes. This is why training in these techniques must be step by step. If you were to study prāṇāyāma with me, I would not mention any of these practices for a long time. Then they would be introduced gradually. What we are trying to develop to bring about unification will, if we move too quickly, divide us into pieces.

Question: When we gaze are we actually using the eye muscles to shift the eyeball position or only using our imagination?

Response: When we are gazing the muscles of the eyes cannot be relaxed. There are effects from different types of gazing. For example, some people are so tense that their brow is always wrinkled. In such cases we always recommend downward gazing, whether on inhalation or exhalation. When the eyeballs move downward, we can't be tense in the forehead between the eyebrows. So to relieve this tension, downward gazing is suggested. On the other hand, gazing at the point between the eyebrows might bring muscular tension. That is why we first gaze at the tip of the nose for a few months before attempting to gaze at the point between the eyebrows. If there is much tension, the technique is wrong. Gazing must be done gradually, otherwise we end up with a headache.

Question: Is gazing for pratyāhāra?

Response: Some people think so. There are texts on yoga that suggest this is the technique for pratyāhāra. But as I explained the other day, we can't establish pratyāhāra, it just happens.

Question: Is candle gazing used only for meditative purposes?

Response: Candle gazing is actually a form of external gazing. We have a convention in India where every morning we look at the sun through a particular position of the hand. The idea is to get used to the form so that when we do prāṇāyāma we can recall that view of the sun. Candle gazing is something like this, but it is not immediately associated with prāṇāyāma. It is sometimes used as an eye exercise. This practice is called trataka. In prāṇāyāma, generally the same principle is used, except we gaze inward rather than outward because in prāṇāyāma the orientation is inward.

XIII

Theory

THE ANTARANGA SĀDHANA, SAMYAMA AND KAIVALYA

I would like to review what we covered in the last theory lecture, the antaranga sādhana. Pratyāhāra was defined as a state in which the senses are not the masters but rather the servants. It is not itself a practice but a consequence of a state of dhāraṇā, dhyāna, and samādhi. We discussed the concept of dhāraṇā as the mind directed towards one point. That is, today we have come here from different places and from doing different things. We have come together and little by little we "click," that is, I start talking and you start following me. What happens is that little by little there is a relationship between what I say and what you receive. For example, at this moment you are able to receive much more of what I say than two minutes ago when we began. I am able to see you and give you what I know about the concepts of dhāraṇā, dhyāna, and samādhi. This is the beginning of dhāraṇā, the orientation of the mind towards one particular object, whether an object in the physical sense or an object in the sense of an idea.

Next we discussed dhyāna. This is the communication between mind and object. I am now talking to you about the subject dhyāna. As I go on, I get more and more ideas about dhyāna and less and less about anything else. This intimate communication confined to one idea or object is dhyāna. As it becomes deeper, the need to think disappears. Things become more spontaneous, not only for me in speaking but for you in listening. A moment arises when I begin to lose my sense of separate presence or individual being, the so-called "I-thing." I am no longer from Madras, no longer an Indian, no longer a teacher, etc. All that matters between us is the subject we are discussing. This is a state of samādhi. In this state of samādhi all that seems to exist is the object, the observed. In this process three events happened. First, I confine myself to a particular object. At this stage, dhāraṇā, there is an awareness of two things: myself and the object. Second, I

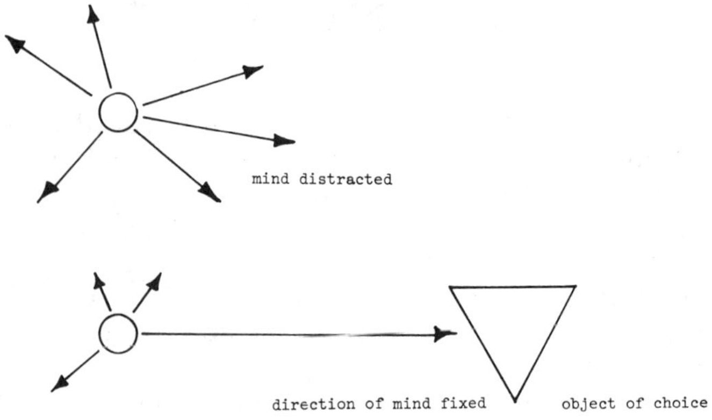

mind in the process of dhāraṇā

Fig. 78

start to investigate this one object. At this stage, dhyāna, there are three things: myself, the object, and the thinking

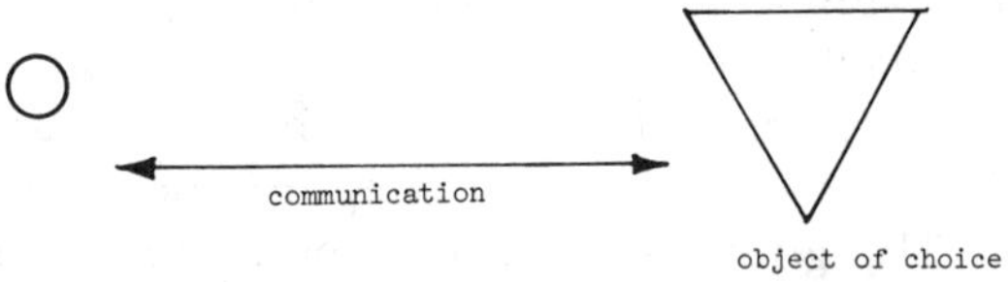

mind in dhyāna

Fig. 79

process or the communication between myself and the object. In dhyāna these three things exist separately; there is a conceptual gap between them. Third, in samādhi there is the intimate meeting of these three as if there were only one. All that remains is a feeling of the object. This ob-

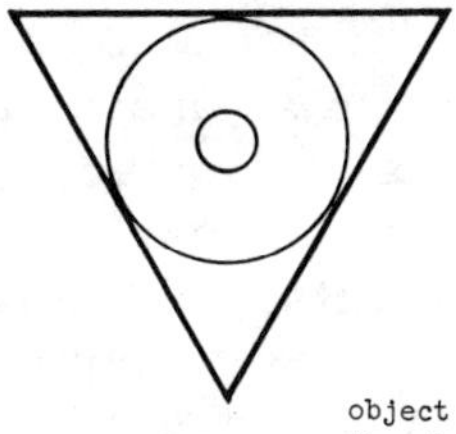

samādhi

Fig. 80

ject of samādhi which we call dṛśya is also called dhyeya which in Sanskrit means "aim." Corresponding to that, draṣṭṛ can be called dhyāta, one who is in the state of dhyāna.

We are not consciously aiming for or striving to do dhyāna. We are really trying to remove the obstacles to dhyāna. We always have a potential for the state of samādhi but somehow something comes between us and that state. This veiling we have discussed as avidyā and its "children." We try to reduce this cover so that this natural phenomenon of samādhi can happen. Anything that aids in removing these obstacles is often understood as dhyāna itself. That is why we have temples, recite mantras, do prāṇāyāma, etc. Therefore, "I am doing dhyāna" really means, "I am trying to prepare myself for the state that is called dhyāna." To say that we are "doing dhyāna" corrupts the word dhyāna itself. So we use the word dhyāna also to mean that which prepares the mind so that the state of dhyāna can happen. There are techniques that might prepare us to move toward the state of dhyāna, and, further on, samādhi. These we will discuss in the course of time.

Question: Could you go over the term draṣṭṛ?

Response: Draṣṭṛ is puruṣa. The word draṣṭṛ means "the one who sees," or "that which sees." It comes from the root dṛś, "to see." So draṣṭṛ is the seer and that which is seen is known as dṛśya, coming from the same root. Dhyeya means "the object of meditation." Dhyāta means "that which meditates." This is the same as puruṣa. Dhyāna is meditation itself. These words, dhyeya, dhyāta, and dhyāna, come from the root dhyai, "to think." This information is only to help you in case you come across these words in the books you are reading. What is important is what they mean. Any questions about dhāraṇā, dhyāna, samādhi?

Question: I'm still not clear about pratyāhāra in dhyāna.

Response: When one gets more and more involved in the object of meditation, one notes, as an effect, the senses behave differently. When I say "object," it is for want of a proper word. Object need not be a concrete object. An object, in this sense, could be whiteness, it could be a sūtra. Please don't take this word "object" in a literal sense. In a meditative state the senses are in accord with the state of dhyāna. They will not distract. Pratyāhāra, then, is an effect of this state of dhyāna. Pratyāhāra is not possible by itself. We can do things that will serve as aids towards pratyāhāra. That is why recently we talked about "gazing" and mudrā in prāṇāyāma, that is, closing our eyes, keeping our hands in certain positions and looking at the tip of the nose so that the habits of the senses are slightly reduced. But this in itself is not pratyāhāra. Pratyāhāra is when the senses serve the mind in the process of dhyāna. To repeat, pratyāhāra is not something we can practice and achieve. It is something that happens in an ideal state of dhyāna. There are certain things we call dhyāna that are in reality only to help us enter into dhyāna like prāṇāyāma, prayer, worship of God. Some teachers also suggest practice techniques for pratyāhāra. They say, "Close the eyes, take a deep inhalation, and send your breath to the toes; exhale then inhale and send your breath to the ankles;" and so on. Actually these techniques are similar to the practice of prāṇāyāma in that the mind becomes less and less distracted. It is very difficult to find a technique for the practice of pratyāhāra itself because the more we use the senses the more they focus upon their objects. All we can do is create a condition in which the senses lose their habitual significance and only help the mind in the state of dhyāna. Is this clear?

Question: In dhyāna, does the object as well as the seer retain an individual, separate identity?

Response: Yes. In dhyāna there is a feeling that "I" am involved in this state of meditation. However, these words have different significance to different people. Sometimes the word dhyāna is used to mean "near-samādhi," that in dhyāna there is only object. I am now presenting these states as a three step progression. First there is dhāraṇā, a focusing on the object of interest by delimiting extraneous distractions. Then dhyāna, communication between ourselves and the object. Third, samādhi, when we are so involved in the object that we seem not to exist.

Question: In samādhi, does the object retain its distinct identity?

Response: Of course. The object is not in meditation, we are. The object might change, as all things change, but not as a consequence of samādhi. What we experience in relation to the object will often be different. Suppose we think about the concept of Īśvara. We read here and there and we begin investigating it. The more we go into it, the more we respond to the concept. It is not because the object called Īśvara is different, it is because our understanding is different. We are able to see something more. We do not change the object, we have no control over the object. Our understanding of the object is different because our minds are clearer so we can see something that we did not see before. The object does not necessarily change; the change is in us.

For example, what is the difference between a state of samādhi and a state of anger? There are said to be four stages in the intensity of the children of avidyā. The first, prasupta, "dormant potentiality," is when they exist as only potential, like a seed. The next stage, tanu, is when they have been extended toward an object, though still mild, like a seed that has sprouted. The third stage is vicchina; here one aspect of avidyā is apparent and others not. The last stage, udāra, occurs when one aspect of avidyā is manifest

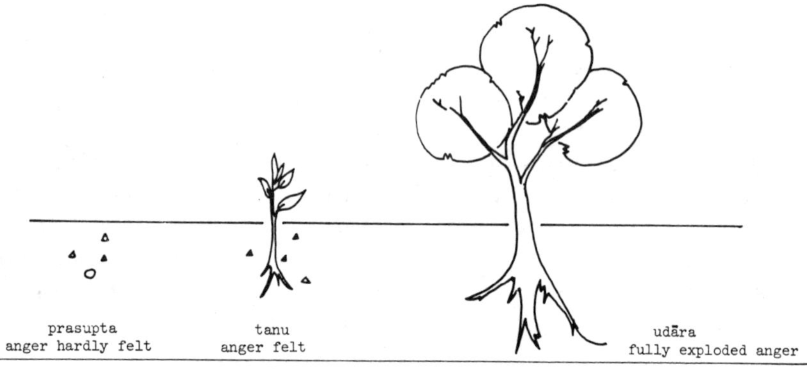

three stages of anger

Fig. 81

and has taken over our reason completely. If we are completely covered with anger it is as if we are not there. All that is there is anger and its effects. Is this samādhi? Can anybody answer?

Comment: I'd say it is not samādhi because in that case, where there is only anger, we are less suited to living easily in the world. In samādhi, hopefully, we would be more at ease in the world.

Response: Good. Very good. Anybody else?

Comment: I would also say anger is not samādhi because the mind is not thinking clearly nor is it in a peaceful state, but rather in a state of anguish.

Comment: Anger at the udāra level is almost the opposite of samādhi. It is not the object that is seen clearly but only the ego. We see only in terms of ourselves and that is how we can be angry.

Response: When a man is at the peak of anger, do you think he is going to see that he is angry? Suppose I have a bad fight with my wife. After a few minutes I am different; I will say, "What have I done?" So, if I see the anger do you mean to say I will remain angry? I would do something to stop my anger.

Comment: I don't think we can see anger.

Response: Just think about it. It is important that we do, otherwise we will tend to overintellectualize this.

Comment: Isn't the state of samādhi something that the individual has some control over?

Response: Control means?

Reply: In anger we are helpless. It just happens to us. In samādhi we are supposed to retain some clarity. We have some control. Can't a person consciously control going into and out of the state of samādhi?

Response: Even anger is a gradual process. It is circumstances that bring anger to its peak.

Reply: But in anger we lose control of ourselves. I would think that in samādhi we would be in complete control.

Response: Anybody else?

Comment: What you just said, that the circumstances bring us to a peak. Isn't that the opposite of samādhi?

Response: Sometimes we practice prāṇāyāma to better prepare ourselves. There are certain things we do in yoga which seem to aid dhyāna because they remove something that is blocking it. If something aids movement toward samādhi, something also aids movement toward anger.

You have given some good points. The answer given in the Yoga Sūtra is very clear. To investigate the nature of anger is a dhyāna. But to be in a state of anger where we have "lost our heads" is not dhyāna. If we read some of the ancient classics, we see that the emphasis is on what happens in the state of samādhi. The state of samādhi is really a state of prajñā. Prajñā in Sanskrit means "clear understanding." In samādhi, ṛta prajñā exists. Ṛta prajñā means "what is seen is true." The true understanding of the object then exists. Even if anger is the object, we see what is anger, how it originates, what are its effects. In a peak of anger, however, we lose ourselves. In such a state, the mind is completely covered with avidyā. Samādhi is when the mind has no avidyā. That is why samādhi enables a person to see something he has not been able to see before. The true test of samādhi is not when we sit cross-legged, close our eyes, and show a lot of nice things on our faces. It is what happens to us, when we see what we have not seen before.

Question: Why is it that as you talk you use the word dhyāna more than the word samādhi?

Response: Because I am able to speak and establish contact. There are systems of meditation in which we are supposed to meditate while walking. While walking something dawns on us and we dwell more and more upon it. Then a state comes where our feet don't move any more, they stop. Similarly, in samādhi thinking stops. In the state of dhyāna there is profound mental activity and communication using the senses there. So if I am talking to you now the "I" is very much present. In samādhi this "I" is very much in the background. How difficult it is to verbalize these concepts!

Question: When a student of yoga begins to experience these things, is it only with the aid of a guru or can he do it himself?

Response: As in anything else, a little guidance is helpful. In theory this seems simple, but there are practical difficulties. There is the choice of an object, where to begin, and how to lead oneself to it. We should always start with something we can appreciate, something which causes us no conflicts. Dare I tell you, because I am from South India, that you must start thinking about Viṣṇu? While this is possible, Viṣṇu might have very little meaning for you. That is why the practice of āsana and prāṇāyāma is very helpful because they demonstrate that in anything we do we must start from where we are, a place of no conflict. That is why we use postures and investigate the breath. Since starting points vary, it is better to find someone for whom you have respect and with whom you have had some contact to help you. This help will give you a little more feeling for the selection of an object. It must not be just an intellectual process. As you know, there are books written on meditation, but how are they going to help you start without knowing you? Any teacher can give you some help because they hopefully can observe you; therefore guidance is needed. The Yoga Sūtra therefore makes no direct reference about going to a teacher, because, at that time, it was taken for granted. Originally the teaching of yoga was passed on by word of mouth before it was finally written. Students would live with their teachers until they got to know them very well. Therefore I feel it is better to have some personal guidance.

Question: It is said that in yoga we try to see the difference between puruṣa and prakṛti. Now you are speaking about samādhi in which the subject/object distinction is absent, there is no gap between them. How do these two relate?

Response: There is no gap but there is observation. I said that we see something we did not see before. Let me again use the example of a mirror. When we are looking into a mirror, we see ourselves. Actually what we see is a reflection in the mirror, not us. Yet in the mirror, the image, ourselves, seems to merge and still we are able to identify these distinctions. When we look in the mirror we can't take out the image of our faces from the mirror without removing ourselves. It is true that at this moment the seer and the seen merge. That means that something which was between them is removed. As I have said, the puruṣa sees the object through the mind. If the mind is colored we are not able to see clearly. When the mind is very clear it is almost as if the mind did not exist. We then see the object as it is. If the object is the concept of prakṛti, we will see it because that which was blocking the observation is no longer there. The problems we have in life come because of saṃskāra. We are not able to distinguish the colored image of the mind from the real object. When I say "I understand" I might think I understand but five minutes later I might say, "Oh, now I am stuck." The same I that thought it understood now feels it does not understand. In the state of samādhi that I is almost nonexistent. The confusion of the mind has been removed. To fully understand this we have to experience it. Despite this, are you able to understand what I mean?

Question: Can there be a state of dhyāna in āsana? Can we use the body as the object and let dhyāna be the communication between us and our body in movement?

Response: Yes. In fact the third chapter of the Yoga Sūtra goes into this. For example, if the object of our meditation is the pole star, we will have knowledge of the movement of stars; if the object of our meditation is on the navel cakra, we will have knowledge of the body. So, yes, it is possible to use the body as the object. If we use the body we will understand more about the body. If we use the breath we will understand more about the breath.

Question: Is a state of samādhi possible in āsana? Wouldn't it interrupt movement?

Response: In āsana don't we have all of the necessary elements: the mind, the object, and communication between them? So what is the problem? It is just that our focusing is different when we do āsanas. If we want to feel a twist, our whole mind orients towards that and we understand what is a twist. In āsana the object of dhyāna is variable. It could be the entire concept of āsana, it could be some detail or special focus, such as a twist, the flow of breath, ananta, or other things. Depending on what we use, what we see in dhyāna will be different. It is often specified what type of object we are to meditate upon and for what reason. That is why in India we have so many gods. If we look at Viṣṇu smiling, we feel one way; if we look at powerful Durgā, we feel another; if we go to Śakti, it is something else. The idea is that the object influences the understanding. This concept is called saṃyama. Saṃyama is when one pursues continuously over a period of time a particular object, one will understand more and more about that object. Suppose we want to understand how the stars move, we have to start pursuing in that direction. So our questions and inquiry will be towards what is a star, whether it moves from east to west, etc. So what happens? In no time we will know more about this object than any other object. That is saṃyama. Saṃyama is dhāraṇā, dhyāna, samādhi, on a particular goal or object over a period of time. Rather than on Monday choosing one object and on Tuesday choosing another, we try to understand completely one particular object without changing our interest. That is saṃyama. If we take as object āsana, we will know everything about āsana. Some say that saṃyama gives us special and supernormal powers. These are just effects of saṃyama and not the goal. To become obsessed with these powers is to miss the importance of saṃyama. To fix upon an object and pursue it until we know everything about it is the goal of saṃyama.

Question: Is it true that every time we learn something we are involved in dhāraṇā, dhyāna, samādhi?

Response: Certainly! It might not be as deep as it is described in texts, but it is the same. If we understand something, our minds must be involved with it. That is dhāraṇā and dhyāna.

Are the states of dhāraṇā, dhyāna, samādhi permanent? It is said very clearly that when a person is in the state of samādhi, there is no other state in him. It is almost as if at that moment he does not remember that he ever had a distracted mind. When a person is distracted, of course, he has only a memory of samādhi. So these states of dhāraṇā, dhyāna, samādhi, on the one hand, and daily confusion, on the other, alternate. A person in samādhi does not recognize that he ever had confusion. A person in confusion might faintly remember samādhi. That's all. In this way, it alternates. As a person gets more and more involved the time for samādhi is more, and confusion less. Eventually a time will come when a person is always in a state of samādhi. We hope for this.

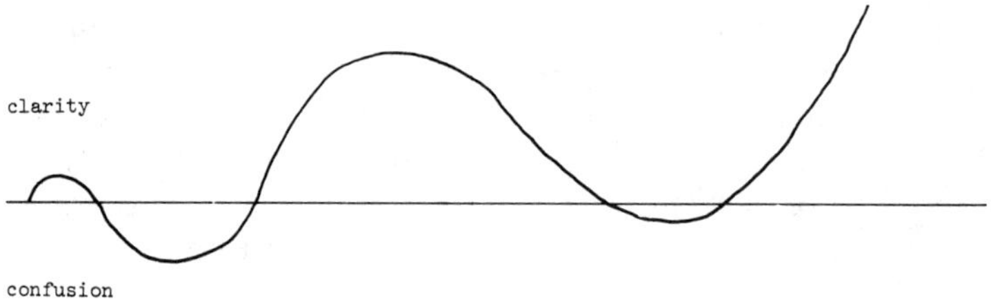

alternating states of clarity and confusion as it progresses

Fig. 82

Question: Is the ultimate goal of yoga to be in samādhi all the time?

Response: The ultimate goal in yoga is that we always observe correctly and therefore, we never act regrettably.

Question: If we are in a constant state of samādhi, how much involvement in the world do we have?

Response: That brings up the next subject I want to discuss, kaivalya. The word kaivalya comes from the word kevala, "to be aloof." It is often translated as "isolation." The state of kaivalya is one in which a person is able to understand this world so well that he is rather aloof, in the sense that he is not influenced by the world though he may influence the world. It is often mistakenly said that a person in the state of kaivalya has no normal functions. In fact, he has all the functions, he behaves exactly as before, but he is not carrying the world on his shoulders. Everything that used to disturb him no longer bothers him. He lives in the world but he is free from the world. But he is not free from the perception of the senses, or the body. He is only a little different. Wherever he is, he is sure of his steps. That is kaivalya. The outside forces that used to influence him so much do not influence him anymore. But he knows the outside world. Kaivalya is the effect upon the whole person the more and more he achieves samādhi.

Question: I remember reading that kaivalya happens suddenly like a breakthrough.

Response: According to yoga, the purpose of the whole creation where puruṣa and prakṛti come together is to provide us with a context for an understanding of what we are and what we are not. When we understand this, there is kaivalya, and prakṛti has served its purpose. To such a person, prakṛti is simply where it is and it has no more purpose. If we do āsanas, gradually we become supple. If we do prāṇāyāma, we gain control over the breath. So, too, with kaivalya, gradually something happens that we do not control. There is always a gap between our effort and these states. There is always this spontaneous thing, something happens in us. As we prepare ourselves for dhyāna properly, the state of dhyāna takes over. I will illustrate with a

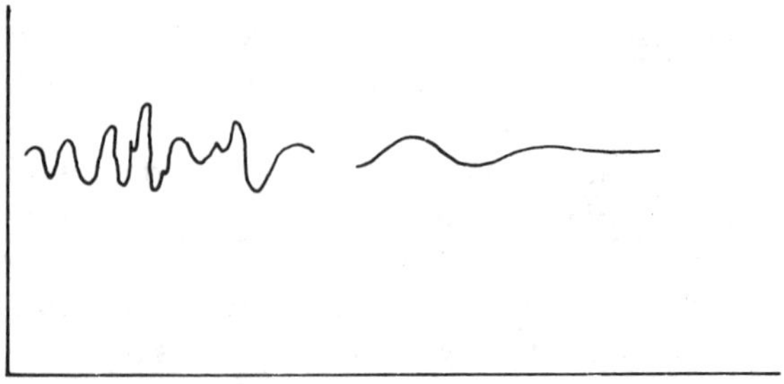

change from distraction to attention

Fig. 83

graph. We cannot discover the moment of dhyāna just as we cannot find the moment we fall asleep. We either miss the moment or we never sleep. In dhyāna we may prepare ourselves but when the moment comes, it is almost a gap or a break, and we are in dhyāna. With the final kaivalya, there is no more oscillation. A person is always in that state.

Question: But then is it a break or something gradual?

Response: We have two forces. One force is our old conditioning and the other is the new conditioning. As long as both forces are operating, the states alternate. When the old force vanishes, there is no longer a question of this alternation. I am not able to say this more clearly because we lack criteria to measure it. How can it be measured? In theory I can describe it as a break or something gradual. At the moment we feel it, what criteria can be used to measure it? Despite this, the Yoga Sūtra describes it as more gradual.

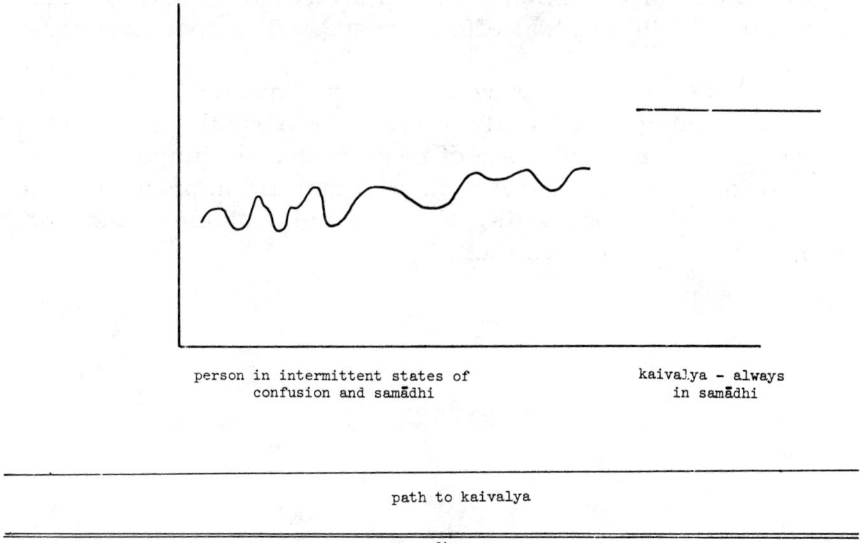

Fig. 84

Question: How does this occur? We can't sit down and practice dhyāna like prāṇāyāma, so how does dhyāna come about?

Response: There is always an effort and this involves two things. While we are trying to do something like prāṇāyāma, there is also something that inhibits us. What inhibits us is really something mental. One force is inclined to practice and the other, old habits, pulls us back. This means that there is necessarily an effort. When the moment comes in which there is no need for effort or trying, at that moment dhyāna occurs. That is why the first chapter of the Yoga Sūtra says we must have abhyāsa. It means, "to go on in a particular direction." The more we go in one direction, the less we will concern ourselves with other directions. Then a moment comes when there is no need to say, "All right, let's do some practice." Suppose I am sitting doing prāṇāyāma and I receive a letter from a friend. One part of me says, read the letter, while the other says, first finish the prāṇāyāma. Because of this oscillation of the mind, there is always an effort. At the moment of _dhyāna_ that effort ceases. It is spontaneous.

In the next lecture on theory (Chapter XV) I will mention the things that really prevent the normal state of _dhyāna_. _Dhyāna_ is a natural state of mind but some things prevent it from occurring. Knowing them might aid in preparing the mind for _dhyāna_; that is, what are the obstacles, and what might help to remove them?

XIV

Practice

THE CONCEPT, PREPARATION, AND TECHNIQUES OF BANDHAS

Today I will discuss bandhas, the theory behind this concept, necessary preparation, and then the techniques.

I have explained how prāṇāyāma helps the fire in the body, sūrya, to reduce the "dirt," apāna. Bandhas are a means by which we can intensify this process. The theory is that the bandhas make sure the flame is brought exactly to where the apāna, "dirt," is concentrated, so that the fire has more effect.

The term bandha means "to bind or to lock." In this process, we tighten certain portions of the torso in a particular way. We will consider just three bandhas: the jālandhara, the uḍḍīyana, and the mūla. The jālandhara bandha involves the neck and upper spine. The uḍḍīyana bandha involves the portion of the torso from the diaphragm to its base. The mūla bandha involves the portion from the navel to the base of the torso. Jālandhara bandha positions the torso in such a way that the spine remains erect, keeping the draft in line with the fire. Uḍḍīyana bandha brings the apāna up towards the fire. Having lifted up the apāna in uḍḍīyana bandha, we use mūla bandha to keep it near the fire. These three bandhas can be used in the practice of āsana and prāṇāyāma. Eventually during the practice of āsana and prāṇāyāma, jālandhara bandha is maintained throughout inhalation, exhalation, and holding the breath. Uḍḍīyana bandha is done only after exhalation is finished and before inhalation is begun; that is, during bāhya kumbhaka, holding the breath after exhalation. As with jālandhara bandha, mūla bandha is maintained throughout the prāṇāyāma. Again, the principle is, make the pipeline straight with jālandhara bandha, bring the apāna toward the fire with uḍḍīyana bandha, and hold the apāna near the fire with mūla bandha. Mūla bandha also blocks the downward

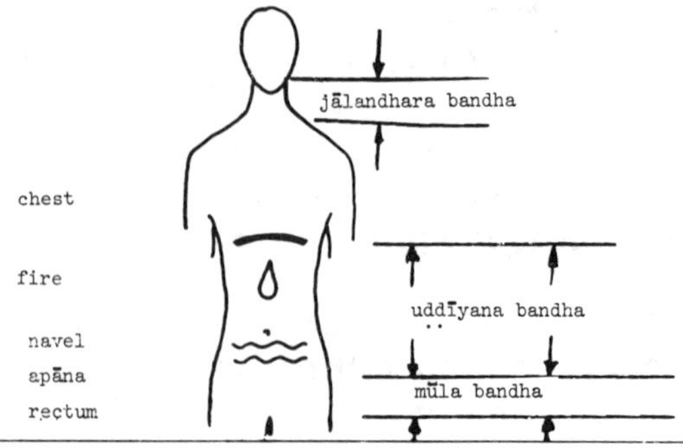

bandhas

Fig. 85

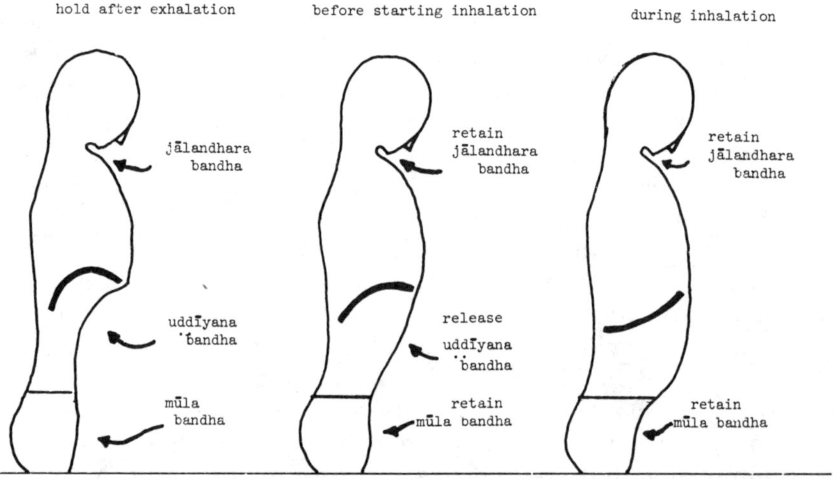

use of uḍḍīyana, jālandhara and mūla bandhas

Fig. 86

movement of prāṇa.

Question: What is the role of mūla bandha?

Response: In uḍḍīyana bandha, we lift the diaphragm and the whole lower abdomen. When holding the breath after exhalation is completed, we release the diaphragm; however, we continue to hold up the lower abdomen. This is mūla bandha. We establish uḍḍīyana bandha and then mūla bandha on the first holding of the breath after exhalation. Uḍḍīyana bandha is then released and mūla bandha is maintained. I will explain the correct technique later.

Now, who is ready to do these bandhas? As uḍḍīyana bandha is done only on holding the breath after exhalation, one of the most important requirements is that we be able to do a long holding of the breath without sacrificing the quality of the inhalation and exhalation. If this is not possible, we should forget about bandhas for the time being. To maintain jālandhara bandha, the neck and back must be in a proper condition to keep the back straight and the chin down. If someone with a very stiff neck tries to force the chin down, he will hurt himself.

We must begin to do these bandhas in some simple postures so that our bodies can get used to them. The easiest posture is to lie flat on the back. We call this taṭāka mudrā when we do uḍḍīyana bandha in this position. Another simple posture is adho mukha svanāsana ("A-frame," dog pose). The next step is to try them in some sitting posture such as mahā mudrā. These bandhas can also be done in the headstand. It is easy to do bandhas in this position because the lifting, uḍḍīyana bandha, and holding up, mūla bandha, of apāna to the flame is almost automatic because now the apāna is above the flame. (Obviously, we cannot do jālandhara bandha in the headstand.) If we can do the three bandhas in these postures, we are ready to introduce them to our prāṇāyāma.

In teaching the technique of bandhas, we begin with jālandhara bandha. If we are not able to do that, we are

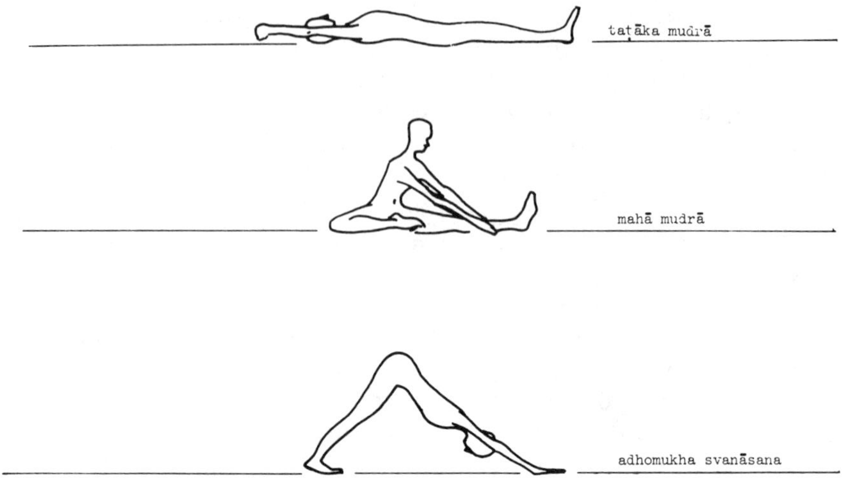

easy āsanas for bandhas

Fig. 87

not ready for the others. In jālandhara bandha, we lift up the back so it is very straight, pull the head back so that it is in line with the spine, then tuck the chin down. In this bandha it is easy to know whether or not our spine is erect. As long as the chin is down and the back is straight, we are in jālandhara bandha. In some postures, this bandha is not possible. (See Figure 86.)

The next bandha we teach is uḍḍīyana bandha. In this technique, as we exhale we start contracting the abdomen. At the end of exhalation the abdomen is completely contracted, lifted, and pulled back towards the spine; at the same time the diaphragm moves upward. If we do this bandha very well, the navel goes back to the spine; the rectal and back muscles contract. At the completion of uḍḍīyana bandha, the whole abdominal area is hollow. (See Figure 86.) I want to caution you that this lifting of the abdomen is to be done very slowly, not rapidly. For example, if we are holding the breath after exhalation for ten seconds, we must take at least two seconds to release the abdomen. If we do not release the abdomen after uḍḍīyana bandha, we will not be able to inhale. We will feel choked. It is very easy to get the feeling of uḍḍīyana bandha in some of the simple postures I mentioned. Remember, this bandha is practiced only after jālandhara bandha is well established.

The mūla bandha is established after we have done the uḍḍīyana bandha. As we release the upper abdomen and diaphragm, we maintain a contraction in the lower abdomen, back, and rectum. That is, the portion of uḍḍīyana bandha below the navel is maintained in contraction while the portion above the navel is released. Once established, mūla bandha is to be maintained throughout prāṇāyāma. (See Figure 86.)

To practice these bandhas in prāṇāyāma we must first establish a ratio of breathing, i.e., inhale/hold after inhalation/exhale/hold after exhalation, that we can do comfortably at least twelve times without the bandhas. Suppose we pick a ratio of 6-0-12-6. I would do the following:

Inhale	Hold	Exhale	Hold	
6	0	12	6	No bandhas for six breaths
6	0	12	6	Use jālandhara and uḍḍīyana bandhas for six breaths
6	0	12	6	Use all three bandhas for six breaths
6	0	12	0	No bandhas for six breaths

The last six breaths of this prāṇāyāma serve as a counterpose. This introduction of bandhas is a very gradual process. As in the daily practice of āsanas, in the use of bandhas we build up and taper off gradually. If we fail in any of the earlier steps, there is no point in going on. This is how we use bandhas in prāṇāyāma.

If we want to do bandhas in the headstand, we follow the same principle. Although jālandhara bandha is impossible, we still can do the others. Any questions on how to do these bandhas, how to build up the practice, how to taper off?

Question: Is there any problem in holding the breath after exhalation for so long in the headstand?

Response: Of course it is not natural to hold the breath after exhalation. We must build up to it.

Question: In inverted postures, isn't the mūla bandha almost a natural effect?

Response: It is not natural though the position aids us in doing it. That's why I said the headstand is a good position in which to introduce these bandhas before we try them in prāṇāyāma. Gravity helps us. But there is a difference between gravity doing it and consciously doing it.

There are obviously some postures in which bandhas are not possible. Normally any posture in which the spine is straight can be used. I did not mention the shoulderstand only because the breathing is rather difficult in that posture. If we can do it, it is all right. We should anticipate a great reduction in our ability to do long breathing and holding the breath once we introduce the bandhas. There is quite a bit of effort involved in doing them. If a person can do 10-10-20-10, I have found that with bandhas the breath is reduced to 6-6-12-6. So don't get worried if your breathing ratio becomes less when using the bandhas.

The best āsanas for doing bandhas are inverted, lying flat, or sitting with the back straight. A classic posture is mahā mudrā, which is, in fact, mahā mudrā only if the bandhas are used.

There are many postures, however, in which the bandhas should not be done, for example, backbending and twisting postures.

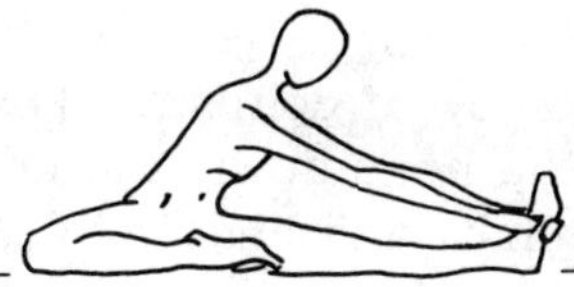

mahā mudrā

Fig. 88

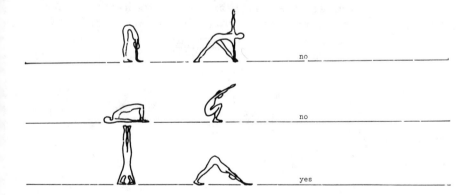

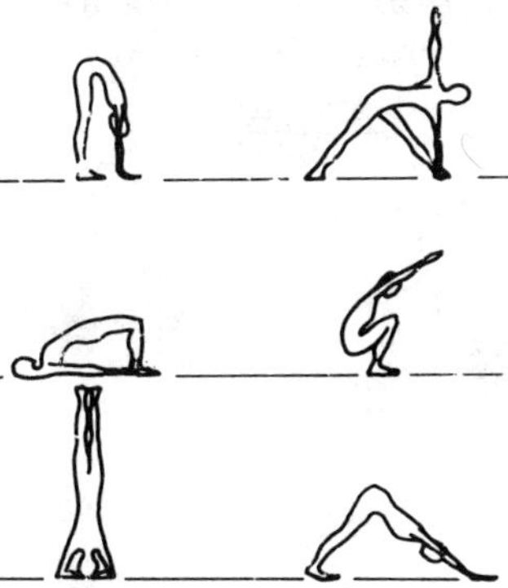

āsanas: whether or not suitable for attempting ba as

Fig. 89

Also we cannot do all of these bandhas in some prāṇāyāma such as kapālabhāti because we don't stop the breath after exhalation. We cannot do them in śītalī either because we are moving the head.

Question: Couldn't we do jālandhara bandha in kapālabhāti?

Response: Yes, of course. That is only one bandha involving bringing the head down and keeping the spine erect. It is used in kapālabhāti and bhastrikā. The other bandhas are impossible.

Question: When we are lying down the back really isn't straight. Can we do bandhas there?

Response: Even though the back is not straight, this is actually one of the easiest positions in which to do the bandhas.

Question: Should bandhas be a part of every daily practice?

Response: Yes, if we are ready to do them. We might do them in any one posture or in prāṇāyāma. Don't do them in all the postures and prāṇāyāma. That will only be negative. Suppose we want to do the following practice:

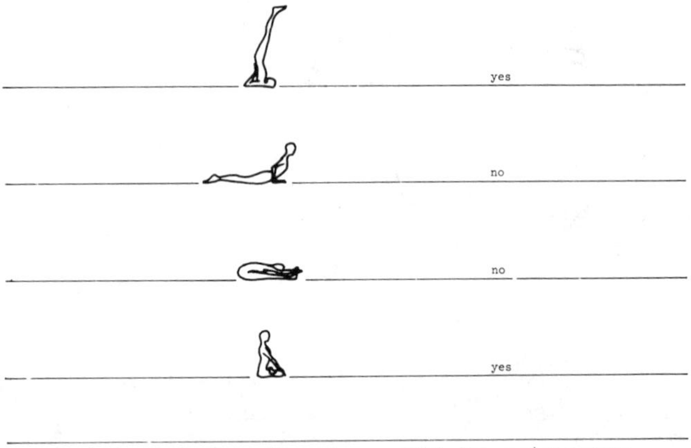

do not attempt bandhas in more than one āsana or prāṇāyāma during a practice session

Fig. 90

In this course we could theoretically do bandhas in two places. I suggest we do them in one of these postures only.

Also there are several positions in which we can do prāṇāyāma. Sitting on a chair, and sitting cross-legged in sukhāsana, siddhāsana or padmāsana. These are the best positions for prāṇāyāma.

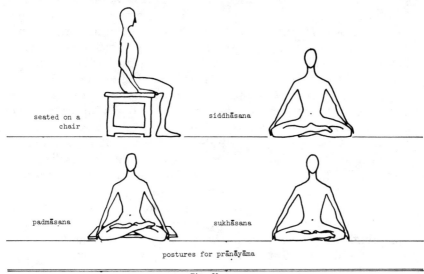

postures for prāṇāyāma

Fig. 91

Question: I read in a book about an exercise of pulling in the abdomen and then at one second intervals snapping it out and pulling it back in, all during holding the breath after exhalation. Is this dangerous?

Response: That is not a bandha. It is called agni sāra. I explained earlier that in a particular context kriyā means "a process by which we clean the body using particular techniques." For example, to clean the stomach a wet cloth is swallowed and then extracted. Another practice is to take a mild salt water solution and pour it through the nostrils in a certain way. When we are doing prāṇāyāma we are using the air and the fire to clean the body. Agni sāra means "fire used as a cleansing process to remove detrimental things." When we are doing any exercise with proper breathing, cleansing is automatic, and other outside means are not necessary. Some people who do not breathe well in āsana use other means.

I must caution you about the use of bandhas after exhalation. Many of our internal organs are involved in the process of contracting, lifting, and releasing. If we don't know what we are doing we might develop some problems. A man from New Zealand came to see me in Madras. He had been doing nauli, a process in which the abdominal muscles and internal organs are moved in a particular way. He thought it greatly relieved his constipation so he started doing it daily six times. Over a period of time he had to increase the number because it became therapy for his constipation. A time came when he had to do it for half an hour and still nothing happened. Then one day he said to me that whenever he ate food his whole abdomen expanded and he had to urinate every fifteen minutes. What had happened was that he had weakened the sphincter muscle which controls the passage of urine from the bladder. It was only after he stopped doing nauli for a few months that he could see a movie without interruption. The body has its own natural processes to clean itself. We just have to encourage that to happen. We shouldn't have to use anything unusual. That particular contracting exercise really isn't necessary because when we breathe properly in prāṇāyāma there is the same effect without strain.

Question: Why must the back be straight for bandhas?

Response: First the back will never be completely straight. The axis of the back must be straight and the spine must be erect, not rounded or hollow. The spine will always be a little hollow towards the base and a little rounded at the top. We want that reduced to a minimum, that is all.

Question: Is it good to change from day to day the position in which we do prāṇāyāma? Say one day we do padmāsana, one day vajrāsana (kneeling, sitting on heels), one day vīrāsana (kneeling, sitting between feet), etc.

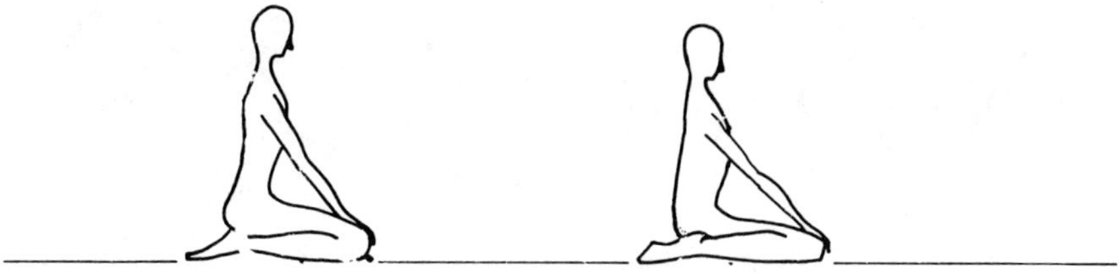

Fig. 92

Response: We can change the pose for prāṇāyāma from one day to another, but we usually prefer to use the same one. We can't use vīrāsana. Who can sit in vīrāsana for long? Also, in this posture our backs are round. In vajrāsana our backs are hollow. Vajrāsana is also difficult to sit in for long unless we are trained as a Japanese kōtō player. We do not advise doing prāṇāyāma and bandhas in either of these postures.

XV

Theory

ANTARĀYĀḤ, OBSTACLES TO PROGRESS: TECHNIQUES TO OVERCOME THEM

We have covered a great deal up to this point. Do you have any questions about dhāraṇā, dhyāna, samādhi, saṃyama, kaivalya?

Question: When you spoke about samādhi, you described it by utilizing a threefold structure: the seer, the object, and the communication between the two. You said in dhyāna the seer and the object merge and there is communication.

Response: They meet and communicate.

Question: You said that in samādhi only the object remains, the seer doesn't matter any more nor does the communication. What happens to the communication?

Response: I tried to make the point that at this stage there is no thought. Thinking is absent in the sense that there is no need to think because we are so much with the object. There is no need to enter a process of saying, "This is like that," "That is like this." We are still present but we understand the object so deeply, so well, there is no need to think, to analyze. This thinking is what I mean by communication. Of course, samādhi has different stages. The samādhi I have just described is more evolved than others where there is still some thinking and communication.

At this point in our program, it might be helpful to discuss an aspect of yoga for those people who want to be a little better but find that somehow they become stuck and can't progress. The term antarāyāḥ describes a situation where a person moving toward betterment is blocked, either because of the experiences had in that progression or because of negative factors that might have been present for many years. Let us consider some of these obstacles, nine in number, how they arise and how to get rid of them.

An obvious obstacle to progress is when we are not well, when we are ill, or have a disease. Of course, we must regain our health. So even if we are ready mentally, and we want to do yoga, to do breathing and to prepare for dhyāna, if we are sick, we must do something about it. It disturbs the mind to such an extent that we have to do something about it before we can proceed.

There is also an obstacle that is from the nature of the mind itself. We get moods--sometimes we are all right, we can go on, but sometimes we feel heavy, we feel dull, we don't feel like proceeding. This mental heaviness could be due to food, it could be due to cold weather, it could be just the nature of the mind. In a previous lecture I briefly mentioned the three guṇas, the three qualities of the mind. One is heaviness (tamas), one is the active part (rajas), and one is the proper state, the whole basis for our work (sattva). When heaviness takes over the mind, even though we are used to doing certain things, we feel so dull that we just don't move.

For some, there is another obstacle, doubt. Suppose we are moving along, making progress, and we have doubts about what should be done next. "Is it worth even five days?" "Should I stop?" "Maybe I should find some other guide or teacher?" "Maybe I should try some other system?" Doubts always arise. There is no doubt about that!

Even more things can happen. Sometimes we act with little deliberation, we want to progress very quickly. Sometimes our actions are done a little hastily and we get into trouble; that is, instead of progress we regress. Due to a lack of analysis, a lack of reflection, our actions, instead of leading us forward, keep us where we are or lead us backwards. So we think we are doing something, accomplishing something, but nothing happens and we become disturbed. This action is without clear reflection and deliberation.

As a result of this action or in spite of it something else might also happen. Because we think our achievement graph is not going up as much as we want or as much as that of another, or as much as we expected, we suddenly get a little dull, thinking, "Okay, maybe I am not the right person," etc., etc. This represents a lack of enthusiasm. In these cases something must be done to regain our enthusiasm and motivate us toward our goal.

Another obstacle is when our senses seem to take over. They reassert themselves as masters, sometimes without our knowing it. This is not surprising since we are trained from birth to look here, see there, hear this, touch that, etc. So sometimes, because of their habitual action of always looking for things, etc., the senses take over and our direction slowly shifts in the wrong way.

The worst obstacle of all occurs when, somewhere in the back of our minds, we think we have understood something and we haven't. That is, we fancy that we have seen the truth. We think, because of a situation in which we feel we have some sort of calmness, we have reached our zenith. We say, "That is what I have been looking for; I have progressed." But in actual fact we have not progressed. This feeling of having reached the top of a ladder is only an illusion. Such illusion is quite common, as when we read a book and because one part of our mind rationally understands something we tend to think very highly of ourselves. We might even think, "I am in this state of sabīja samādhi."

The next obstacle finds us in a situation in which we presume we have progressed a lot, but in reality, when we deal with society, we find that we have much more to do. We become rather disappointed, indeed, we become fickle. Instead of going forward, we just stop; that is, instead of reaching the goal in yoga, to understand more and more and more, somewhere in the process we say, "No more for me. I thought I got it but I think now I am like a fool, in fact worse than others, so I just don't want to do any more." We just stop. These are eight of the nine different ways obstacles can come. As you can see, the obstacles can be as simple as a physical disease, or as subtle as illusion; that is, we think we are somebody better than we really are. When we work on this basis, when we become aware of illusion and come face to face with reality, we feel, unfortunately, we are really a little less than what we are. This can create our last obstacle, a situation in which we reach a point that we have never reached before, but we are unable to stay there, we allow ourselves to slide back. So, at every stage, we must never think that we have become masters. There is always a sense of being a little better than yesterday and always, too, a sense that we can be a little better tomorrow. This movement remains present until we reach a point where there remains neither a better nor a worse. So these are the obstacles in the progress of yoga. They do not necessarily follow one after the other.

Further, just as yoga identifies a number of obstacles that stand in the way of progression, so also yoga provides alternative ways or methods to surmount those obstacles.

The most important method given to surmount obstacles is the concept of Īśvara-praṇidhāna. This is submission to Īśvara, and it springs from great devotion and belief that there is some spirit higher than ourselves. We pray to him in our own way, believing that he does and will help. With greatest faith we leave all our efforts in his hands and we proceed.

Īśvara is apart from the material, prakṛti, and the seer, puruṣa. The qualities of Īśvara are many: in brief, he sees things as they are, he acts perfectly, he is all-knowing, the first guru, a source of help. Īśvara, unlike us, is not influenced by avidyā, he is beyond avidyā. Although he knows what avidyā is, he remains uninfluenced by it and therefore he never acts wrongly, he has never acted wrongly, he will never act wrongly because he has never been covered by avidyā. In fact, because he is never covered by avidyā, he is able always to see things that we are not able to see. Therefore, he should be a means of guidance for us. Further, Īśvara performs no actions that bring about negative repercussions or regrettable effects. For him, there is no vicious circle of action, bad effects and their conditioning leading to bad actions, bad effects, and further bad conditioning, etc. He is beyond this circle, of which he is aware but by which he is not influenced. Like puruṣa, he is also able to see; he has the quality of seeing. That is why the Yoga Sūtra says that he is a puruṣa, but a viśeṣa puruṣa. Viśeṣa means "extraordinary." He is extraordinary in the sense that he has no avidyā, therefore he has no evil, regrettable actions, no duḥkha. Moreover, because Īśvara is beyond avidyā and duḥkha, he has a potency within himself that enables him always to know everything. In yoga, the word for this quality, a word also used in other systems, is sarvajña. Sarva means "all," jña means "to know." "All-knowing" means he knows everything always, at every level. And this quality is restricted to him, it is a quality that we as human beings don't have. So Īśvara has no avidyā, he really sees, he is beyond error in action, and, as a consequence, he is sarvajña, that is, he always knows everything.

Because of this he is the master, venerated because he is the guru. He is the guru because he knows everything, and since he always knows everything, he is the first guru. Because he always knew, he always knows, he always will know, he is the pre-eminent guru. So our respect for him is because he knows and so we pray to him, "You know, share with us your knowing."

Yoga does not describe Īśvara in a particular form. To have a relationship with him, yoga uses a special symbol to represent him. This symbol is called praṇava. Praṇava is OM. According to the Yoga Sūtra the way we contact Īśvara is through OM. We recite OM with the idea that OM means Īśvara. The more we continue to recite this symbolic sound, while delving into the meaning, the more we gain an idea of Īśvara. In this process, the mind, instead of being distracted, merges into this symbol and concept. At this moment, we become quiet and we can begin to progress.

What is our relation with Īśvara? We accept him

totally as the final teacher to whom we pray, in the hope that he might help us because he can help us. Īśvara, then, is one of the alternatives suggested in the Yoga Sūtra for surmounting obstacles. I am not able to find an English word for Īśvara; perhaps it is "God" or "Lord" or something else. Please be patient with me because I don't know quite how to put it.

Question: You said after class one day that yoga is the inversion of prakṛti and puruṣa, so that, instead of the world being on top and against us, puruṣa is over the world. So puruṣa controls the senses rather than the senses controlling puruṣa. If one is going to give oneself over to the protecting guidance of Īśvara, then what does the puruṣa do? How then can puruṣa be the master?

Response: In this situation puruṣa is not our master, that is why we go to some other master. Suppose we are trying to better ourselves and somehow, somewhere we find ourselves stuck. We need help. The only help we need is a little more balanced mind, a little more clarity of mind, because when there is clarity of mind, we progress, no one has to push us. At the moment when we are stuck, maybe we should try prāṇāyāma, maybe we should do āsana, etc. That may be enough. But yoga offers alternatives, and foremost among them is devotion, faith, and complete trust in Īśvara. The question you raise relates to a conversation the two of us had. Let me now share with all of you the point of that conversation that this question addresses. Although in creation, the highest aspect is puruṣa, then the mind, the senses, and finally the body; in life this relationship is gradually reversed. The puruṣa is pushed down. Over it rules the mind, over the mind the senses, over them the body, and finally "the outside." Yoga aims to reverse this process. The real quality of the human mind, the human creation, is such that puruṣa is chief. But what tends to happen is confusion. Puruṣa becomes buried, we don't even know where or whether it exists. Gadgets and the outside world become the boss. Yoga attempts gradually to bring back our real nature, where puruṣa is the master, followed by the mind, the senses, and the body. Therefore, all below puruṣa are meant to serve it.

Question: If all these things are meant to serve puruṣa, is puruṣa meant to serve Īśvara?

Response: In yoga, the question phrased this way does not arise. There is no relation of service as such between puruṣa and Īśvara. What I am trying to explain is how, when a person has confusion, when a person is going in a path of improving himself and at moments he is not able to progress, something can be done. If a person thinks he needs guidance, he needs a little space in the mind. One of the things that can be done is to pray to the Lord, as you say, to have complete devotion and faith in that called Īśvara, the one who is beyond all avidyā. Perhaps, by thinking about him, delving into him, our minds will be more relaxed and become clearer. Whether puruṣa is going to serve Īśvara is not at issue.

To continue, the reasons for the choice or use of OM as an audible symbol are very interesting. OM is a sound that is very much respected in India and in cultures heavily influenced by India. There is Om Maṇi Padme Hum, Om Nārāyaṇa, Om Nāma Śivāya, and the like. OM is always present in these mantras. With the sounding of OM, we are saying everything. Upon analysis, OM has four aspects. The first is "A" (pronounced "ah"), which comes from the abdomen and is formed in the open throat, with the mouth opened. The second part is "U," formed in the middle of the mouth. Then, with "M," the lips meet, and the mouth is closed. The sound then moves into the nasal cavity, so something else is there: (1) "A," (2) "U," (3) "M," and (4) something else. We don't just say "O" plus "M." There are four aspects that together form OM.

"A" in Sanskrit, as well as some other languages, is the first letter of the alphabet. "U" represents a continuation and "M" is the last of the alphabet. So "A" to "M" through "U" represents the entire alphabet and whatever can be represented by letters. When conceived as all words it is a representation of Īśvara. Further, the extended sound after "M" has no particular designation like "A" or "U" or "M." So whatever the alphabet can represent, and whatever the alphabet cannot represent, that too is Īśvara.

Something that cannot be explained by words is also Īśvara.

Moreover, when we say "A," we open the mouth and this opening stands for creation. "U" stands for the continuation of the creation. "M" represents the completion, the dissolution. "M," in a sense, means I have to stop and close my lips, but then there is more, a continuation of sound. Therefore, all that is created, all that can be created, all that is sustained, the power behind creation, subsistence, dissolution and beyond is also Īśvara. It is also said about OM that "A" represents a waking state (as if yawning upon awaking). "U" is a dream state, and "M" is a state of deep sleep. The fourth state is called samādhi. This analysis points to the one who is the master of all these states; there is only one who is awake. That is Īśvara. In the "A" state, maybe we are awake, although yawning. In the "U" state we dream, but we don't know how we dream or what dreams we dream. And in the "M" state, the state of deep sleep, we are not even present. And beyond? Of course, this we do not know. But there is one who is always present in all these forms because he never sleeps, he never dreams, he is always awake, and he knows and is beyond. Therefore, Īśvara is properly represented by OM. So when we repeat OM with these concepts in mind, very gradually we delve into this, and our minds get so absorbed that they become still. After this we can again proceed. That is why Īśvara-praṇidhāna, that is, this way of devotion to Īśvara, complete faith, and delving into his meaning is also one of the ways we can remove the obstacles that come as we progress in life.

I want to remind you that this is only one of the alternatives for removal of obstacles; yoga does not insist that you accept Īśvara. If you find this concept meaningful, continue with it. Otherwise consider other alternatives.

Question: If I were to try chanting OM, should I have, must I have an idea of what Īśvara is?

Response: When we say OM, the meaning must be Īśvara; Īśvara is beyond avidyā; he who knows, who knew, who will know, who always knows. So, if Īśvara can guide us, we think we can become better. It is a form of meditation where we utilize a process of mental reflection on the particular concept called Īśvara. Since Īśvara is beyond the natural forms that we can appreciate, we need a symbol and that symbol is OM. And what is OM? When we say OM, we think of OM as representing Īśvara. Each time we recite this sound, we must allow some time so the mind starts thinking about what the sound represents. So, both repetition, called japa, and its meaning, called artha, must be present. Otherwise our chant will be just mechanical, parrot-like and this will not help. It might be of help for the first few days, but not later. The meaning is important because the more we go into the meaning, the more new meanings we will find. Therefore, there is always new discovery. So japa, repetition, and artha, meaning, are both involved.

There are other alternatives that might help us to overcome obstacles, to keep the mind steady. Some people might not find Īśvara-praṇidhāna particularly meaningful. For them it is important to find something else. One alternative is to find a means that will enable us to sustain a particular direction of discipline. Suppose we have one particular teacher we follow. Sometimes with him we hit upon something new only to find that it leads to nothing. Our immediate urge is to go to some other teacher, and then to still another, and so forth. The Yoga Sūtra says we are not to do this. We are to try to keep the same relationship, one that will lead to deeper communication and trust. When I trust my teacher, really trust him, and when he discovers this trust, even if he does not know what I should know, he will find out what I should know. By following one principle, one teacher, one discipline, we find a means to avoid or surmount obstacles.

Prāṇāyāma is often mentioned as an alternate way to help surmount obstacles. When we are a little disturbed, prāṇāyāma, particularly with emphasis on exhalation, is suggested. This is called recaka prāṇāyāma, where we inhale normally but make the exhalation very long and pause after exhalation. So even simple things like breathing also help.

Investigation into the functioning of the senses can also help us calm our minds in order to overcome obstacles to our progress. We can investigate how the tongue functions, how it tastes things at the tip, in the middle, and in the back. Such investigation quiets our minds though it greatly depends on the individual. It is not the discovery of the way the senses function that is so important. Rather, in that moment when we are stuck, the mind is given a little space.

It is always important that when we are stuck, we must stop struggling to move. We should never try to force progress. How, then, can we set about to prepare to progress anew? We need to give a little space to the mind. So we pray to Īśvara, we do prāṇāyāma, we try to have more contact with a teacher, or we investigate the functioning of our senses. When there is confusion, we must find some space in the mind.

Another alternative is suggested for those people who accept a concept that deep in the body, somewhere in the heart region, there is something called the puruṣa. The Upaniṣads state that there is a small muscle in the region of the heart, and that deep within it is a small opening like a lotus bulb. Inside that is a small space and in this space is the puruṣa. It is always glowing there. Inquiry into this concept often brings the mind to quietness.

One of the best ways to remove obstacles is to study people who have overcome a lot of problems (duḥkha) in their lifetimes. We will discover, as we read their writings and find how they have solved their own problems, that which might also help us. In India there are very many temples, each with stories of its founding, explaining its location and its tradition. When we go to a temple, we ask about the sculpture, the symbols, who did what, and often we are told moving stories. We come to see the way the symbol relates to us. We come to know that it is real. As we go more into this discovery, our minds find some freedom. This also helps us to progress. There are many of these stories in all religious traditions.

When we find we are distracted, it is often helpful to investigate something that constantly happens in us, but about which we know very little. We could investigate how dreams come about, what is the concept of dreams, who is dreaming, etc. We could examine sleep, what is sleep, what sleeps, and how one awakens. We could even study how it is possible for life to continue. If we calmly seek knowledge about these things, it will help our minds to become quiet. Investigating dreamless sleep might be helpful because deep sleep is an example of a state in which unconsciously we have the most peaceful life. That is why this sleep is called suṣupti, "deep sleep" (good and healthy). Some people say that in sleep we the children, the puruṣas, are sleeping in the lap of the father, Īśvara. So by investigating sleep, what dreams are, and how we dream, we can also bring the mind to a state of quietness. Not only do we discover a little more about sleep, but also we feel better, enough to proceed.

Suppose we are not particularly interested in pursuing any of these alternatives. We can attempt a form of meditation that utilizes a visual object. That is, we can reflect on something we find meaningful. Take, for example, meditation incorporating the use of an image of a deity. While visualizing this image we repeat the name of the deity one hundred and eight times, one thousand and eight times, or some traditional number that relates to the particular deity. We delve into the concept of the particular deity: Who is Śakti? Who is Śiva? Who is Viṣṇu? This activity is preparation for dhyāna. We make an attempt to meditate, we try to be with the image of the deity. We describe him with poems that have been written by great poets, we repeat his many names. This type of meditation also helps the mind to become quiet. We have to use such objects for meditation that bring a quality of peace to the mind. We cannot use those objects that stimulate mental distraction. So even though we have great freedom of choice, we should always select those objects that suit us and that definitely bring a state of quietness. Although the Yoga Sūtra says one can meditate on anything of one's choice, it means anything of one's choice that one knows brings the mind to quietness.

There are many ways we can get over a situation in which we become stuck and can't progress. When we are stuck, for whatever reason, we can always find a solution, some means to overcome our obstacles. Perhaps, now you can appreciate how open yoga is to alternative procedures.

Question: Can you elaborate on what you mean by "give the mind some space"?

Response: "Space" means freedom at the moment when we are stuck. When we are stuck, there is no space, there is no freedom. That's all.

Question: Suppose we are trying to get over some obstacles to achieve a quiet state of mind in relation to the concepts of yama and niyama. I'm wondering whether Īśvara might be more suitable in view of yama; that is, our participation in society. If we have this complete devotion, this complete faith in relationship, as opposed to just breathing, a long exhalation, etc., wouldn't it be more of a personal sort of activity? Wouldn't Īśvara aid the overall betterment of the individual?

Response: If I understand your question, you are asking, "Is it possible to say that devotion to Īśvara is better than the other alternatives?"

Reply: Yes.

Response: The answer depends upon the individual. If a person comes to me and I say at the outset, "Why don't you pray," I might not be addressing the person where he is. Some people hate this very sentence. "Don't try to tell me to pray," they reply, "I don't care for Īśvara." Where should I begin with this type of person? I was like that. When I took my first reading with my father, who is my teacher in the Yoga Sūtra, I told him, "Don't preach to me about Īśvara now. I want to know about yoga. I don't want to be taught how to pray." While I would not say this now, I did then. As I mentioned on the first day of this program, we have to give a person what he is prepared to take, not necessarily what is finally best for him. So, no matter how good it is that people accept Īśvara, some just don't care about this notion.

But later, automatically it seems, a respect comes. I've found through experience that for many people, who had the same view as I had when I took my first lessons in yoga, something happens. I don't know why; we seem to respect some force or higher presence called Īśvara we would never have accepted before. This always happens; this has happened to people in all walks of life, but we can't lay it all out in the beginning. No, we can't put a block in communication by insisting on something. This openness is something very important in yoga. That's why in yoga everything is real but things change. So when a person is ready, we'll talk about Īśvara.

XVI

A SESSION FOR QUESTIONS

In our previous lecture on theory, we discussed obstacles that might arise in the course of one's progression in yoga and alternative ways to overcome them. I am sure that you have many questions. I am prepared to spend the entire session today responding to your questions.

Question: When there is difficulty, is it possible or useful to direct attention to that difficulty, rather than to get into all those different ways that you suggest? Sometimes focusing on the difficulty could be helpful, it seems. One could learn a lot from that.

Response: Suppose I have a problem with my wife, should I investigate this problem rather than do the other things? This question points to a helpful distinction. If we have a problem which persists, it might be because we don't know what is the real basis or cause of the problem. In terms of yoga, if we have duḥkha, something is behind it. So if I have a persistent problem with my wife, it is really because I don't know the real basis of the problem. If I go on thinking and acting as if the problem were money or something else which it is not, it will only become greater. The best thing would be to develop a state of mind where we really see the whole thing afresh. There might even be no problem. Maybe I just think there is a problem. So, if we do something that clears the mind enough to see deeper than what we believed was the problem, the problem might become more manageable or disappear.

Reply: But when we do something like this, when we change our state of mind or whatever, it seems that what we now see is not the same thing as that which we wanted to look at.

Response: Say I do something that will make the mind become a little clearer. At that moment I will not be looking at the problem. There is a "gap" for the mind, a few moments in which the mind is not pressurized by the problem. Consequently, when I again turn my attention to the situation, I see things differently. The problem is different and when things become different, it is not because something deep in me has become different, it is because more external things have become different. Because the "I" has become different, the stress of the problem, the intensity of the problem changes. Now, perhaps, I can solve it. Who knows what might happen; the solution depends upon the individual. But my suggestion is to develop a state in which the mind becomes lighter and is able to see something much more clearly. Something that was acute might become less acute because our priorities might change. What we thought was most important might no longer be the important thing. Perhaps the problem can then be solved.

Question: In the grip of a problem, isn't it hardest either to sit or to be quiet because the one who is trying to make the mind quiet is the one who is frustrated?

Response: In the beginning this is true. That is why when we are gripped with a problem, yoga suggests we try to change our environment. Get out of the place. Go somewhere where something else acts rather strongly on us so that our problem is behind us for a while. For example, think of something else, go to a movie, or just do something. This is a step preceding the step of quieting the mind. The first step is a sort of escape, but sometimes even escape works. Even solutions to our problems are sometimes suggested by something within ourselves or something not in our consciousness. This is why a certain evolution is required. The more we are in this process of evolution, the more we find solutions by getting away from a problem, not because we want to avoid problems, but in order to come back afresh and sort it out. We need both incidental solutions and continual progress. That is why yoga suggests that we move stepwise, from incidental solutions to continual progress. When you see these two steps act together, you will understand why sometimes even escape is good.

The idea is not merely to run away, but to step away and to return so that we can see things in a different perspective. From the perspective of pariṇāma-vāda, of yoga, the mind and everything outside the mind is always changing. What we then need is a little time. With time, if we can find it, we become a bit different so we see things differently. We are no longer in the state of having an acute problem.

Question: Relating to this, there is a sūtra which says that avidyā and the things that proceed from it, hate, likes and dislikes and all that, can be reduced by resolving them back to their origin. I don't really understand what it means to trace ignorance back to its origin.

Response: This sounds like a poor translation of one of the sūtras. Sometimes we seem to have no problem. Things go well, we get our money and we have things, everything is fine. During those times it might appear that we don't have anything that can be classified as avidyā. So this sūtra cautions, "Don't think there is no avidyā. Get on with it, get on with it!" because you never know when avidyā might quickly arise. "Resolving back to the origin" means to be in a state where avidyā is no longer effective. It is like taking a seed from the soil, removing its husk and burning it--the seed becomes useless. "Resolving back to the origin" also means to put something in a state where it is no longer effective. Even though we don't have an immediate problem it does not mean we will never have a problem. For example, one day I started playing cards with some friends. I was really glad because I had not played cards for many years. They said I played well. Suddenly, you know what can happen in a card game, I got the wrong cards, or I'm not sure I know what happened, but I got all the bad points. My score was zero and so was I! These things happen. We never know when or how, so we must be cautious. To be cautious, we must keep on trying; that is what abhyāsa is all about. Abhyāsa means constant effort and attention in order to continue in one direction. We must never break this process because we never really know in advance how things might change. Through abhyāsa, we carry on, without interruption, for a long time until the seed of avidyā is burned. Once there is an interruption, detrimental processes can arise, even when our intentions are good and loving. Abhyāsa may be developed through the practice of āsana, prāṇāyāma, self-study, or an attempt to move towards meditation. But we must keep on developing this ever-present effort and attention because we never know when avidyā can appear.

Question: When you spoke of obstacles that get in our way, one of them was a lack of enthusiasm or loss of enthusiasm for doing yoga and other things in our daily life. What in particular helps us to regain that enthusiasm? What can we do?

Response: What we need is greater effort to go in a particular direction. This is the fundamental concept of abhyāsa. We lift ourselves up with sheer effort to stay in the direction we have chosen because we believe it is good. So naturally when we attempt this, since we have old habits, there is always something that drags us down. That is why, once in a while, it is good to go to our teachers. In their presence we might regain our enthusiasm. It is also a good idea to read books about this. We can talk to people who are enthusiastic about our interests. Yet another solution is just to accept fully what happens and when we are low enough, we will find strength to do something about it. When a man is really sick, he will usually find medicine. These are the two kinds of solutions: somehow, if we are able, we lift ourselves up; or we accept our lack of enthusiasm until we get so many problems that we have to go forward again. I think the first one is better than the second because in the second one we may become so confused that we don't know where to go and therefore, we tend to make mistakes. That is why mental effort is required. Are there any questions about the notion of Īśvara?

Question: You said one should devote oneself to Īśvara with complete trust, with faith. In this devotion and faith, does Īśvara then control us? Can Īśvara make us see the truth, or something like that, because Īśvara takes control of what happens?

Response: Yes, if we completely trust Īśvara. We must have some conviction about Īśvara. This conviction is deep within us. We must feel that there must be something that is called Īśvara. We may define it in any way we like. This conviction can come in three intermingling ways. The first way, the most difficult but the best, is to have seen Īśvara. Obviously what we mean by "seeing" is not the seeing with our eyes. We recognize somewhere deep within us that there is something higher than ourselves. Another way we conceive of Īśvara is by inference. For example, some people say that if the stars can always be above us without falling down, there must be something that is holding them. We are not doing it. Other people are not doing it, it must be something higher than ourselves. It is Īśvara. This is one way people infer the existence of Īśvara. Another way this conviction can come is through the testimony of textual authority and the testimony of people we trust. These, then, are the three ways that lead us to the acceptance of Īśvara: directly, indirectly, and through textual or scriptural authority. If we have complete trust in Īśvara through any or all of these ways, we can progress. But if we have doubt, we will not. Even so, sometimes from doubt we can discern faith in Īśvara. We never know. We start with doubt, but somehow we go on solving problems and we see more and more that there is something higher than us, and we can then accept Īśvara. But simply invoking Īśvara might not suffice; we have also to do something. So conviction is very important. For those people who don't have this conviction, Īśvara cannot help, at least in the beginning.

Question: Does Īśvara control everything?

Response: What do you mean by "everything"?

Reply: The whole world.

Response: Yes. In yoga, our concepts are a bit different. According to yoga, Īśvara knew, knows, and will know; he is the first who knew. The whole creation has two aspects: the material and the intelligence. Suppose we make a pot. What do we need? We need clay, of course. We also need water, fire, a potter's wheel, like they did in the olden days. We also need someone who can make the pot. That person is the one who recognizes that a pot can be made, that water is needed, that a perfect mound has to be formed, that there needs to be a wheel and the clay must be worked this way and that. So for every creation we need at least two things: material and intelligence. The material is the clay, the intelligence is the potter. In yoga, material is not from Īśvara, but intelligence is. Everything that is created, how it has been brought about, its relationship to other things--everything has behind it the intelligence, the wisdom of Īśvara. He is the intelligence behind all creation and all motion. He may not be the material itself because, just as clay can't make a pot from itself, material cannot shape itself. This is the way Īśvara has been conceived and venerated in yoga. He is the one who is the intelligence, the sustenance, everything behind the whole creation.

Question: Could you look at creation as having three necessary parts? One could be material, one could be intelligence, and one could be the force of the wheel, or something like that.

Response: Yes, we have this notion in yoga. While I didn't want to elaborate unnecessarily, we do have three things. They are called kāraṇa, "a means for something, a cause." For any creation we need three kāraṇas. One is upādāna, material. The second is nimitta, intelligence. And the third is sahakāra, assistance. To repeat, the nimitta kāraṇa is Īśvara.

Question: Much earlier you were talking about a certain detachment that is needed in normal life so that we are not totally blinded by avidyā. Is that detachment not also necessary when one is trying to focus all one's attention on an object of meditation?

Response: In a sense, yes. But that detachment is an effect, a consequence of another deeper action. For example, a temple is a place where we can be in a particular atmosphere while looking at a beautiful image. The more we look at it, the less we will be interested in other surrounding things. In this case detachment is the absence of attachment to any other objects except the image of the god. Detachment can also be the absence of attachment toward the fruits of what we are doing at the moment. The more we get involved in this process of communication with this image, the less we see it as stone, as an idol. It represents something else, other, deeper things that automatically follow.

There is a beautiful story that might serve as an example. Once there was a lady who was married for ten years, and still childless. She went to this temple and that, she gave a cow and many other offerings. Finally, she was told to go to a pipal tree, which is often used for praying. She was told to go around this tree one hundred and eight times every day and that in the course of time God would help her. She was naturally delighted. So she went there and did the usual things; offered a coconut, betel leaf, etc. She kept going round and round and round the tree until, after one hundred times, she felt her abdomen to see whether she was with child. She was not as much involved with prayer as she was with the hoped-for effect of prayer. In fact, she was not praying. This type of activity represents the opposite of detachment. If you are completely involved in prayer, automatically there is detachment and surely, automatically things happen.

So detachment is automatically the consequence of deep meditation, devotion or prayer.

Question: Concerning dhāraṇā and dhyāna and thinking in terms of Īśvara being the object, how would you describe the mind in the state of being one-pointed in dhāraṇā with Īśvara as the object, moving progressively toward dhyāna?

Response: Objects can be different, and, on the basis of which object is utilized, the state of mind is different. Suppose I have a look at Michelangelo's statue of David in Florence. My whole state of mind becomes different because I see the human body. I reflect upon the beautiful figure. All the memory that I have about the human form comes before me. So my state of mind is one of beauty because that statue of David is beautiful. Now, suppose I look at Śakti, who is so ferocious, with her thousand teeth, her frazzled hair and those vicious canine teeth. The more I look at Śakti, the more I develop a state of mind which is really terror. So, depending on the object of meditation, the state of mind changes. If we have an object that is very peaceful, very kind, replete with compassion, healthful, then our state of mind becomes like that. In this way, the state of mind changes according to our concept of *Īśvara*. If we consider the concept of *Īśvara* as the one who is the most intelligent, who is the wisest, who is the intelligence behind all creation, who has no *avidyā*, our state of mind will resemble that. In this case, because the object of mediation has no *avidyā*, the process of meditation also has no *avidyā*. That is how *Īśvara* has been so conceived because, when we meditate through prayer or the repetition of a *mantra* to him, gradually *avidyā* is reduced. So naturally the object influences the mind, depending upon the description of the object and upon the memory that we have of the object. That is why when we look at the Buddha, everything that is Buddha, the compassion, the serene love is present in his face. When the sculptor does his work well, and we really look at the Buddha, the mind also becomes quiet.

Question: I am not clear about the relation of *dhāraṇā* and *dhyāna*, one-pointedness in concentration, and the notion of one being intermittent and the other continuous. How do you mentally concentrate on *Īśvara* in light of these stages or phases of concentration?

Response: I think the definition of *dhāraṇā* must be refined here. Suppose I have a hundred things on my mind as I sit here before you. *Dhāraṇā* comes when I orient my mind toward one idea, one concept, one object. *Dhāraṇā* is not an interruption of *dhyāna*, that is, first *dhāraṇā*, then *dhyāna* for two seconds, and then an interruption, followed by *dhāraṇā* for two seconds, another interruption, etc. *Dharānā* simply is a state of *ekāgrata*, one-pointedness of mind. It is when the mind, instead of ramifying outwardly, converges toward a particular concept or object. That is all *dhāraṇā* is. When this happens, *dhyāna* should follow. As examples of the process, in *dhāraṇā* I say, "I'm going to investigate the concept of *Īśvara*. What is *Īśvara*? This is what the Yoga Sūtra says. This is what that man says. How can that be? This is nonsense! How can somebody who has no body do something?" This process is the beginning of dhāraṇā. Then gradually as I see a little deeper, I become involved with the Īśvara concept, and the link between Īśvara and me becomes profound. This is dhyāna. Then as I get more and more into the process, I see something about Īśvara that I had not seen before--and that is samādhi.

In a sense, it could be said that dhāraṇā can be intermittent, but it is more accurate to speak of it as having the possibility of being interrupted by distractions. Dhyāna is a bit more continuous in the sense that we become more steadily involved in this activity. It is important to note that the clear demarcation that might appear as we list these processes in discussion are not so clearly drawn in practice. Very generally, we say that in dhāraṇā, we go in one direction of inquiry; in dhyāna, we communicate with the object, and in samādhi, we are there, we are with it.

Question: In this process of dhāraṇā and even in the beginning process of dhyāna, isn't it the "ego-mind" that consciously stews about a concept and, for example, the different aspects of Īśvara or different relationships with Īśvara, like submission or distraction? Isn't this actually the activity of the "ego-mind" and not puruṣa?

Response: True. But what is this "ego-mind"? Apparently you have some idea of what it is?

Reply: Asmitā.

Response: What else can there be in the beginning?

Question: In dhyāna is it asmitā which is communicating?

Response: Yes.

Question: Some of the solutions you suggest to eliminate or overcome obstacles could be seen as symbols by which we discover more about them and about ourselves. I sense that a symbol endowed with mystery can be much more effective in achieving dhyāna, than, say, contemplating the life of Aurobindo or others. What are the implications of choosing, say, an object of meditation that doesn't have mystery? I suspect that discovery would not be maintained and there would be more of an opportunity for distraction. Mystery always draws us on, whereas if we are just contemplating, say, on breathing, there might be too much habit possibility there. Do you get a sense of what I mean?

Response: I have really got it. What is mystery? Mystery is where we always have something that we cannot understand. Do you agree with this brief definition?

Reply: Yes.

Response: Now, how can we say there is no mystery in breathing or in the story of Aurobindo. We might start studying the story of Aurobindo. We don't know at the outset where it is going to lead us. It is not that we are going to get stuck with historical details: where he was born, where he lived, etc. That is just the beginning, the first step. Say he next talks about integral yoga. What is integral yoga when yoga itself is integral? We might wonder about this concept. In this way we can go on and on, yet Aurobindo is always somewhere in the background.

Something similar can occur if we were to consider Lakṣmī. In the beginning we would probably see Lakṣmī as simply a beautiful woman with no flaws in any of her features, as though a sculptor had created a form in near perfect proportions. That is the first step. But we don't continue looking at Lakṣmī as a beautiful woman. We might ask, "Why is she called Lakṣmī?" There is the mystery here. And further, "Why does she have a hundred and eight names?" "And what are those one hundred and eight names?" In this way the story begins to unfold. It is a similar situation when one considers breathing. What is it that makes the breath go in and out? Is it simply breath? We can go back to praṇa and beyond. Mystery is always present; it need not be limited to symbols or God. It can be found in anything, provided we seek it. It is in the hands of the seeker, not in the object. Mystery is always there, everywhere, provided the seeker is serious.

Question: You mentioned earlier, with regard to yama and niyama, that as one progresses gradually changes happen. That also seems to be sort of what you said about dhāranā and dhyāna; they just happen.

Response: "Happens" does not infer that we simply do nothing. We have to try. We must try. We have to try something that seems to bring us a sense of wholesomeness within.

Question: Then what about self-denial, where the scriptures say it is good for us yet we don't agree?

Response: What is self-denial? Please explain that for me.

Reply: Suppose we want to eat meat and we read somewhere a passage that says we should not eat meat. Although we want to eat meat, we don't eat meat.

Response: If we don't eat meat and we don't worry about it, it is all right. But if we say, "I didn't eat meat, I didn't eat meat, I didn't eat meat," and we start dreaming about it, there is no self-denial. In fact, this causes an even stronger feeling about the self rather than denial. It is better to eat meat.

One of you raised a question with me the other day and I have been waiting for it to be raised again today. Since it was a good question, let me repeat it. "The day you were explaining things that might help to reduce obstructions you said that one thing that might help was that we should stick to one thing, one discipline, one principle. Is it not possible to do many things and to integrate them, like, for example, to practice Zen, to do prāṇāyāma, and to worship in church services? If I can integrate them all in my life, isn't this all right?" What is the answer to this question? Is it all right to follow a practice where we combine different convictions, principles, and concepts; for example, Zen, prāṇāyāma breathing, going to church, even fasting, and other practices? That is quite a few. If we combine them and integrate them, is it all right? What is the answer? Feel free to comment.

Comment: As long as there is a sense of discovery, as long as we keep on discovering and growing it is all right.

Response: Anyone else?

Comment: It seems that as long as there is no contradiction or no tension between any of them, and there is no undoing of one by the other, it would be all right.

Comment: If we are to follow only one principle then the integration of different practices can become that one principle.

Response: Any other comments?

Comment: Is it possible for one person to overextend himself? We can try so many different things and in the process lose the point of each one, just by trying to do them all.

Response: In my view, it seems that if a person has the capacity and the means to integrate these things in such a way that one of them does not work against the other, as one of you suggested, it is all right. But if a person has this capacity and means, I don't think he needs so many different systems. One is sufficient as long as there is an openness to investigate. After all, it is good to investigate what the Bible says, what this or that tradition says, but to incorporate them all as a means to remove obstacles is satisfactory only if you can bring a cohesion between them. Some people will go to California for a yoga lesson with a particular teacher, and then to New York for another. The man in California says you should never breathe in postures, it is dangerous, so they never do the breathing exercises there. The man in New York, like me, says "no breathing, no yoga, you must work on breathing or get out." How can you really practice yoga with this conflict, unless you are doing it merely as exercise? You would have to give up both and begin again, or give up one of them. But if you have the capacity and are strong enough to integrate them in such a way that one does not work in conflict with the other, it is all right. I doubt very much whether a person with this capacity to integrate needs all these different practices as long as he continues an inquiry into the system in which he is progressing.

Question: Regarding inquiry as it applies to the self, that is, self-inquiry, I can see how I can come upon things that I am not, but I don't really understand how I can really find what I am. Because if I am consciously inquiring into myself, isn't that an act of my "false self" anyway?

Response: This is something like a kōan in Zen. We get stuck when we think we know the answer. We say it is this way or that. But we begin to grow when it dawns on us that the answer is not found in this way, it is not "in the head." For example, when a svāmi asks us to inquire into the question "Who am I?" and we stop at an answer like "I am a boy," or "I am prāṇa," or "I am Indra," we are finished. The point of self-inquiry and therefore your question is to lead ourselves beyond "I," to see and to cease "I-questioning." All this means that whatever I can recognize with my mind as the greatest is not really the greatest. The greatest is something beyond this recognition. To emphasize this, we ask, "Who am I?" because that "I" is such a variable. We ask, "Who am I?" because the "I" stops at the moment we find the answer.

When we are confused, when asmitā is there and avidyā is present, how can we discriminate between the real and the nonreal, how do we know what is real and what is not real? That is the concept of asmitā and avidyā. When we confuse the unreal with the real and the real as the unreal, we cannot discriminate. Therefore, we have to find other means. Among other things, we do breathing and meditate, because at the moment when the mind is very clear we can see. It is like a clear ocean with no waves, we will see the bottom clearly. The more we try to discriminate, to "work with the waves," the more obscuration occurs, the waves increase. We can never see the bottom this way, we only see the waves and bubbles.

Question: What happens to the puruṣa when the body dies?

Response: That is difficult because we don't have the answer in the Yoga Sūtra. It never mentions death. It does mention fear and some commentators say fear is present because man has died; therefore, he has the fear of death. But this is only one viewpoint. A comment at the end of the Yoga Sūtra might be relevant. It says that when a man has seen what he is, he just stays aloof and is not disturbed by anything outside of himself. While yoga does not answer this question, there are answers provided in the Hindu tradition in general--one of these likens death to many rivers all going to the great ocean. But I don't know, really, because I am answering your question without direct experience. Any answer would be an intellectualization. Please excuse me.

Question: When you were giving different ways of overcoming obstacles, you suggested that one of the ways was by investigating a situation that regularly happens but is not well understood. In that context, you mentioned dreams. What do you mean by investigating dreams? Would it be remembering a dream and thinking about it?

Response: One of you introduced the notion of mystery into our discussion, and did so very beautifully. There is some mystery about dreams. It is not easy to dream and for that matter it is not easy consciously to try to sleep. There is some mystery about this. It is a mystery that we can attempt to explore. This is why it is suggested we investigate how we dream, what brings about dreams, how they happen, why we see certain colors, etc. Sometimes we might discern through this investigation something we have never seen before. Is there not a little mystery about dreams? Once we begin to investigate something we become involved with it, and the mind becomes calm and quiet. That is the idea.

Thank you very much for your fine questions.

XVII

VARIOUS APPROACHES TO YOGA

This is the last day we have to discuss the practice of āsana and prāṇāyāma. Let me begin by asking whether you have any questions?

Question: I find that while practicing āsanas my attention wanders from what I am doing. Do you have any suggestions?

Response: First I would suggest that you vary the āsanas you use from day to day. If you still have this problem you might try to fix the length of inhalation and exhalation in your postures. This practice will surely bring your attention to the postures. For example, try to inhale six seconds and exhale eight seconds in bhujaṅgāsana. Many people have this problem of maintaining attention during practice. You can place your attention on a particular part of the body but there must be something happening, a movement. That is why the best movement is the breath. Those of you who have been doing yoga for some time can fix the length of inhalation and exhalation reasonably and try to maintain that ratio throughout the movement in a particular posture. The ratio you choose will depend, of course, upon the posture.

Question: Could you suggest a book which we could follow that would help us continue to progress after our course together is over?

Response: I would not suggest a book. I'm sure you can find a teacher or even have some correspondence with someone who knows both you and something about yoga. That would be better than trying to follow a book. Different books start in different ways, so where are you going to start the book? I have told you that books are no substitute for a teacher. The best thing is to follow a guide. Even with what you learned in this short time you can always find something new, even in the same practice. As

I have suggested, modify the breath in postures. Don't put too much emphasis on the number of postures. That is where you will end up if you follow a book. It is not that all these postures are useless, but they are not the only way of investigating through yoga. You can discover something new in the same posture by modifying it, fixing the breath, etc. One day I spoke about the many ways to bring attention to the postures. I'm sure this procedure is the best way. Don't go on doing a lot of postures; if you do, I think the meaning in yoga will be lost. There are some postures that might be good, which suit a particular need. It is best to consult a teacher to learn them. You know some people are so supple that they can probably master any position they see in a book, but what does that mean? It doesn't mean anything. Some postures are necessary and for them you must seek guidance. After that you must be on your own.

Question: How do you use praṇava and japa in prāṇāyāma?

Response: First you must learn from someone who knows and who is willing to teach you. You will be taught a particular way to recite OM orally, how much time you have to spend on the first part of the mantra, on the second part, the third part, and when and how to taper off. One day I mentioned briefly these four aspects. I think once you know how to recite the praṇava orally you will be able to do it silently. And perhaps each time you can add a little meaning to it as well as find a little more meaning in it. The best way to learn is to begin orally and then transfer it to a mental recitation. Then you can easily use it in your yoga practice.

Question: I read that you are supposed to count the praṇava in sevens in prāṇāyāma?

Response: The number of times you say OM on inhalation, holding the breath, and exhalation is influenced by the length of breath. We cannot fix the number of recitations on the basis of the praṇava itself. We can only fix it on the basis of a person's capacity of breath. If you are simply using OM, it can go with almost any ratio. If you are using something more complex, say the gāyatrī mantra, it is very long and has different structures so there are regulations on how many times you say it when you inhale, hold the breath, and exhale, and in what part of the mantra you can break, etc.

Today I thought I would enumerate some things you might come across when you read different books on yoga. We have not spoken of the various approaches to yoga and their special emphasis. Yesterday I had an occasion to talk informally with some of you; I was asked if I exclude haṭha yoga from my yoga. Somebody might also ask, "Are you doing rāja or laya yoga?" I thought it would be useful if I defined some of these approaches. While it does not relate directly to our practice, some of the meanings are very instructive. There are about eighteen used in the Bhagavad Gītā alone. Let us consider the following: jñāna yoga, bhakti yoga, mantra yoga, rāja yoga, kriyā yoga, karma yoga, laya yoga, tantra yoga, kuṇḍalinī yoga, haṭha yoga.

Jñāna yoga. Some people say that dhyāna is the means to jñāna yoga. In this context, this means inquiry about the truth, the real understanding that we attain in a state of samādhi. So inquiry in which first we hear, then we reflect, and then gradually we see the truth, is jñāna yoga. In the Yoga Sūtra it is said that in the state of mind where there is no avidyā, automatically there is jñāna. The "truth seeing" that happens in the state of samādhi is jñāna. That jñāna is always there. Jñāna arrives automatically when something that is blocking it has been removed. That is, we want to understand something about X, and by using different means we gradually become completely involved in X. We become X. At that moment there is complete jñāna about X. Jñāna yoga is where we hear or read somebody's words, delve into them deeply, discuss them with people, engage in reflection, until finally all doubts are cleared. We see the truth, we merge with the truth, and that is jñāna.

Bhakti yoga. Bhakti comes from the root bhaj

which means "to serve; to serve that which is higher than ourselves." I have already explained this in the context of Īśvara-praṇidhāna. By any means, we serve the Lord whom we believe is the final source of guidance and help. Serving means many things. In whatever way we act or think, we are acting and thinking for him. In whatever we see, we see the Lord. For example, I can't be aggressive towards someone because I see in that person the truth that is Nārāyaṇa. My relation with people will completely change. To see in everybody the highest truth, to believe we are working for him in all our actions, to think always of his name, to meditate on him, to go to his temples, to show great devotion towards him is bhakti yoga.

Mantra yoga. A teacher who knows us very well might give us a mantra which has a particular connotation because of the way it has been arranged. If that mantra is repeated in the way it has been instructed, if we are aware of its meaning and if perhaps we want to use a particular image, mantra yoga brings about the same effect as jñāna or bhakti yoga. If we respect the teacher who has given the mantra, and if we respect the concept that is behind the mantra, we will have complete trust in the mantra and nothing but help will come from it. The derived meaning for the word mantra is "that which protects the man who receives it." The mantra is not something we find in a book or something we buy. It is something that is given by a master only after great deliberation, after knowing us and knowing our interests and needs. Otherwise a mantra will not be effective. While it might have some effect in the beginning, it will not last. To be effective it must be received properly and repeated over a long period of time.

Rāja yoga. The word rāja means "the king who is always in a state of bliss, who is always smiling." In this context rāja could mean the Lord that I mentioned in bhakti yoga, that is, that something in us which is higher. Also when we understand the truth of Īśvara that is rāja yoga, the Lord will become rāja. Any process through which we achieve greater understanding of that which appears mysterious and obscure in the beginning is rāja yoga. In the Vedas there are many references to the word rāja in relation to Īśvara.

There is a definition of rāja yoga for those who wish to understand it without relating it to Īśvara. In each of us there is a king, puruṣa. Due to our actions, past and present, the puruṣa is suppressed. That is, in a person with confusion and misery the puruṣa is suppressed by the mind which is fed by the senses, reacting to the hundreds of objects that they are constantly serving. Because of avidyā, puruṣa is pushed so low that it is almost as if it were not there. When this process is reversed, where puruṣa ascends to its true place, it is established as king. Puruṣa is the master and all other things serve him. That is called rāja yoga. In both cases, rāja yoga is that yoga where the king, whether puruṣa or Īśvara, assumes his proper place. This meaning is very close to the Yoga Sūtra that states where there is no confusion, the puruṣa prevails and sees. This is rāja yoga.

Kriyā yoga. Much can be said about the word kriyā. We have already discussed in detail kriyā yoga as the yoga of action, that part of yoga we can practice. Therefore, all the practices indicated in yoga are kriyā yoga. Some of these practices are āsana and prāṇāyāma.

In Patañjali's Yoga Sūtra, second chapter, first sūtra, it is described as consisting of tapas, svādhyāya, and Īśvara-praṇidhāna. Tapas are practices such as āsana and prāṇāyāma to aid in the removal of physical and mental impurities; svādhyāya means inquiry and questioning; Īśvara-praṇidhāna is to leave the results of our actions at the discretion of the Lord.

Recently kriyā yoga has become popular in the context of what is called kuṇḍalinī. I will describe kuṇḍalinī later in detail.

Karma yoga. Karma yoga, so very important in the Bhagavad Gītā, is given the same definition as Īśvara-praṇidhāna in the Yoga Sūtra. We have to do our duty and doing our duty is itself more important than what we aim at getting from doing it. We can only act. We cannot be sure of the fruits of our actions because there is somebody higher than us who knows what is right for us. We must act in life, but we should not be disappointed by the results of our actions for we may often act imperfectly. We must act completely and leave the rest to the Lord. That is the concept of karma yoga. This is similar to kriyā yoga.

Laya yoga. It is best to explain laya yoga in a context of samādhi. When the puruṣa completely merges with the object of meditation, that is laya. Laya means "to merge." We merge with the object and nothing else exists.

Tantra yoga. This yoga has been given many meanings and there are many disputes over these meanings. Tantra yoga involves special techniques. To realize what is called yoga, emphasis is placed upon kuṇḍalinī, often described as a coiled and sleeping serpent at the base of the spine. When kuṇḍalinī is aroused, its movement is directed to different centers or cakras along the spinal column.

To understand kriyā, tantra and haṭha yoga properly, we must first go into the concept of kuṇḍalinī which applies to all three.

One of the accepted concepts behind kuṇḍalinī is that we have certain passages in the body through which prāṇa can enter and leave. These passages through which prāṇa can enter when they are free from impurities, pass through the trunk and intersect at six points: at the eyebrow, at the throat, somewhere in the middle of the heart, at the navel, just above the base of the trunk, and at the base of the spine. These passages, called nāḍis, criss-cross throughout the trunk, one starting on the right side and terminating on the left and the other starting on the left side and terminating on the right. As you recall, when there is avidyā the prāṇa extends beyond the body. We make an effort to change the state of mind through prāṇāyāma and other means so that the prāṇa can enter and be totally inside the body. According to this concept this takes place through two nāḍis. There are many names for these nāḍis. They are called ha and ṭha, as in haṭha yoga, which are the names of two small gods; or they are called iḍā, left, and piṅgalā, right, which are just proper nouns.

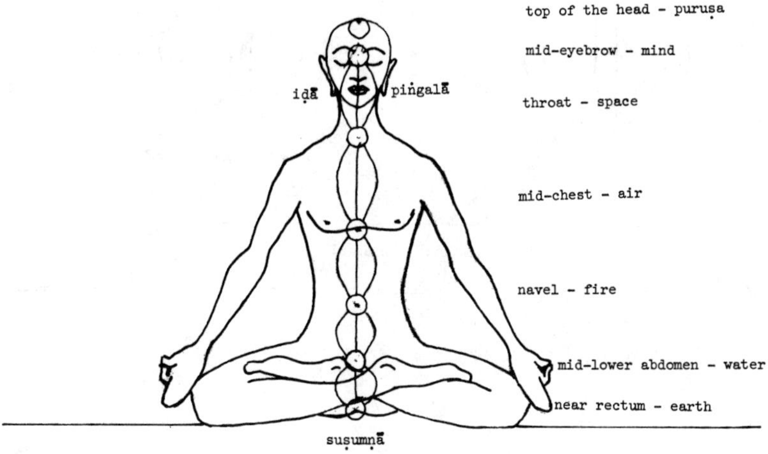

body divided according to the cakras and the travel of the important nāḍis

Fig. 93

Figure 93 shows that even though these nāḍis criss-cross, there is a central nāḍi, called suṣumṇā. Normally the prāṇa enters only in the iḍā and piṅgalā nāḍis. In yoga the ideal position for the prāṇa is in the suṣumṇā. When the prāṇa is in the suṣumṇā, it is not outside the body. If it is not in the suṣumṇā, it is because there is an obstacle blocking its passage. That obstacle is represented as a coil. What is normally happening is that the prāṇa is in the ha and ṭha (iḍā and piṅgalā) nāḍis. If somehow the prāṇa enters the suṣumṇa, the ha and ṭha become one. That is, the prāṇa of ha and ṭha unite, the word yoga meaning here "to unite." That is called haṭha yoga.

The obstacle is called kuṇḍalinī because it looks like an earring worn by women in the olden days and

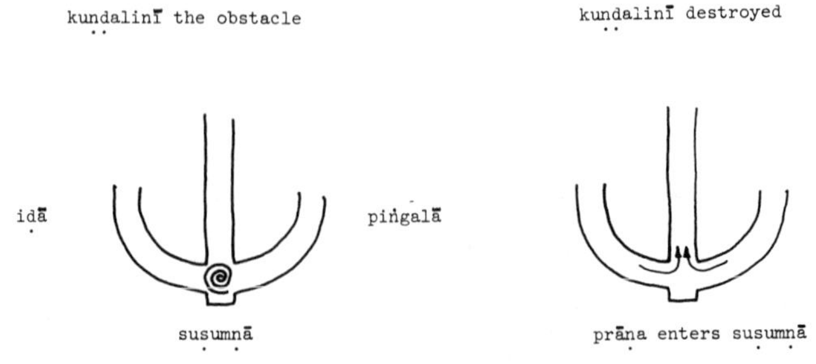

location of kuṇḍalinī

Fig. 94

kuṇḍali means "earring." It is also called Śakti because its power is so great that it is able to block the flow of *prāṇa* into the *suṣumṇā*. We must note that it is *prāṇa* that is eventually supposed to go into the *suṣumṇā*. Many books describe that which goes up as *kuṇḍalinī*. *Kuṇḍalinī* does not go up. *Suṣumṇā* is like a conductor through which energy flows. This energy is the same energy that is always present, *prāṇa*. In this context, *bandhas* are an attempt to direct the fire or heat of the body in order to remove the *kuṇḍalinī* bit by bit. That is why the spiral concept is suggested. Even though parts of it are slowly removed, still the *kuṇḍalinī* has the potential of blocking the *suṣumṇā*.

In *haṭha yoga* one means suggested for the destruction of *kuṇḍalinī* is the *bandhas*. If you analyze what I have been saying, you will see that *kuṇḍalinī* is nothing but what has been called *avidyā*. In the same way that *avidyā* has become so powerful that it stops *puruṣa* from seeing, *kuṇḍalinī* blocks *praṇā* from entering the *suṣumṇā*. The moment *avidyā* is not there is the same moment that

shape is distorted when part of it is sheared off
shape is retained even if a part is removed

difference between a circle and a spiral

Fig. 95

kuṇḍalinī is removed. Then *prāṇa* enters the *suṣumṇā*. As it enters it rises slowly to the top. That is why this is also part of *rāja yoga*. *Rāja yoga* is the process in which the *praṇā*, which is the friend of *puruṣa*, little by little ascends to the top and then the man is like a king, a master.

This movement is also called *laya yoga* because *praṇā* returns to its original position, the *suṣumṇā*.

It is called *kuṇḍalinī yoga* when the emphasis is given to the concept of *kuṇḍalinī*. It is called *haṭha yoga* when the division between *ha* and *ṭha* is removed. It is also called *tantra yoga* when certain energies which are normally spent elsewhere can be used in such a way to help reduce the obstacle that blocks the *prāṇa*. The techniques that operate here are special and so the word *tantra* is used. *Tantra* means "technique."

Sometimes *mantras* have a beneficial effect in removing obstacles. If we look at Figure 93 we can see that

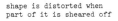

the body has five parts, each related to one of the elements of prakṛti. The throat represents ākāśa, space, because we need space to be able to speak. The heart is vāyu or air because prāṇa is there. The navel area is agni or fire. The lower abdominal area is ap or water and the rectum is pṛthvī or earth. Added to these are two other representations. The eyebrow is the mind, sometimes called buddhi, sometimes citta, and other names. The highest position, the crown of the head, represents puruṣa. Together these seven things make up the cakras. Each represents one of the five elements, the mind and puruṣa. In some books each cakra is given a beautiful notation. For example, the navel cakra is represented by the syllable rum because fire is represented by rum. The throat cakra is represented by the syllable hum. The study of these sounds and the notations attached to each of these cakras have been made into a very elaborate science. By placing our attention on these cakras, becoming involved in this concept and following certain practices including mantra given by the guru, we can remove obstacles. Finally, what it all comes to is that avidyā, here represented as a coil, must be removed. The coil has been compared to a coiled serpent. If we kill a serpent which is coiled, the coil will straighten. A dead serpent is always straight because the muscles no longer hold the coil. It is said when the fire in the body is used to kill the serpent, the kuṇḍalinī straightens and the passage for prāṇa is clear. The kuṇḍalinī has been destroyed. (See Figure 94.)

Question: Does the same thing happen in the other yogas? That is, when one becomes a jñāni for example, and avidyā disappears, is there some physical experience corresponding to the removal of the kuṇḍalinī? Is kuṇḍalinī a representation of an idea or a physical reality?

Response: It is real as are all other things. In yoga there is no question of the unreal because the unreal is also the real. Your question is how to represent this in the case of a jñāna yogi. Ajñāni means "one who does not have jñāna." Jñāna means "true and correct understanding of things." When there is a wavering mind, jñāna is not there. The terms ha and ṭha also represent two extreme sides of a wavering mind. *Ha* often is meant to represent the sun, *tha* the moon. *Suṣumṇā* is the middle *nāḍi* (see Figure 93). *Prāṇa* in *ha* and *ṭha* represents a confused and wavering mind. *Prāṇa* in *suṣumṇā* represents a clear, steady mind. Hence, *jñāni* is one whose *prāṇa* is in *suṣumṇā* and *ajñāni* is one whose *prāṇa* is still in the opposite two *nāḍis*, *ha* and *ṭha*.

Question: So the same process occurs when *avidyā* is removed for both a *jñāna yogi* or a *bhakti yogi*.

Response: Yes. Only different schools represent the process differently. Many of these descriptions are obvious and explicit in the *Yoga Sūtra*; however, *ha*, *ṭha*, and *kuṇḍalinī* are not mentioned. The *Yoga Sūtra* looks at all this in a more fundamental way. It is mostly concerned with a state of mind. Whatever happens to the state of mind happens to the whole person. That is the basis in the *Yoga Sūtra*. In various yogas, the same thing is stated in different ways, that is all. The results are the same because these are merely interpretations of the same thing.

Question: I have read that when *kuṇḍalinī* is released, it is like a powerful electric shock going through a wire. If the wire isn't heavy enough to carry the current, it burns out. So they are saying it is dangerous and we must be prepared.

Response: What is the danger? It has to be described this way because there is some mystery about it. The mystery is that we can't rip open our bodies and see this power. If we relate it to the *prāṇa*, there will be no mystery. My explanations are based on what I think is the best, classic and most straightforward text, the *Yoga Yāgñavalkya*. I think the explanation found in it, as I have given it to you, is more coherent than any other I know. There is no shock here. When a person sees the truth the only shock is that he sees he was a fool before! There is no question of 440 volts or anything like that.

People often ask me if I teach *āsanas*. When I say, "Yes, I do," they say, "Oh, you are a *haṭha yogi*." If I talk about the Yoga Sūtra they say, "You are a rāja yogi." If I say I am chanting the Vedas they say, "You are a mantra yogi." If I just say I practice yoga, they can't understand. They want to put a label on me. Unfortunately these classifications have become too important in all societies and give the impression that in various forms of yoga things are all different and unrelated. They are all the same, only different perspectives. There need be no confusion. If we pursue one direction it means we are pursuing every direction.

Question: Is the use of bandhas the exclusive means for removal of kuṇḍalinī according to haṭha yoga?

Response: No. If you read the Haṭha Yoga Pradīpikā by Svātmārāma Svāmin you will see that there are no exclusive means. He offers different ways in different chapters. The same is true with the Gheraṇḍa Saṃhitā, Śiva Saṃhitā and other classic texts. It appears different. That is why these things must be made clear by someone who knows both the subject and the language. Otherwise there will be confusion. While it is used as a metaphor that the kuṇḍalinī is going up, really, it does not make sense. If we say kuṇḍalinī is an energy that gives us truth, then we have to accept the fact that we have two energies in life, prāṇa and kuṇḍalinī. Some also say that energy is sleeping. What is meant by this? Many of these ideas, I'm sorry to say, are based on incorrect translations. Kuṇḍalinī represents avidyā, and absence of avidyā represents absence of kuṇḍalinī.

Question: When we burn kuṇḍalinī little by little, is there a little more prāṇa entering the suṣumṇā each time?

Response: Yes, that is the idea. It is as I told you about the state of mind one day. Sometimes we have the state called dhyāna or samādhi, and sometimes we are in a state of distraction. In the state of distraction, kuṇḍalini is coiled and blocks suṣumṇā. When the mind is more steady, kuṇḍalinī is not blocking it. A state may arise when there is only one state of mind. Then one is always able to see clearly. That means the prāṇa is going higher and higher in the suṣumṇā.

Question: Could you explain laya yoga again?

Response: Laya, in this context, is when the prāṇa is in suṣumṇā, not outside it. Laya also means when in a deep state of meditation we merge with the object of meditation so much so that we don't seem to exist at that moment. Laya means that two things merge. The Upaniṣads say when we add salt and water, where is the salt and where is the water? Can you differentiate? That is laya.

XVIII

Theory

THE WAY THE MIND FUNCTIONS AND THE CONCEPT OF NIRODHA

Today I would like to talk briefly about the way the mind functions and what is meant by nirodha. The mind functions at five levels. Mostly it functions in such a way that we hardly notice it. So much happens, so many ideas, perceptions come and go that very often we lose track. It is like a monkey that is drunk and somebody is poking it. It is distraught and cannot comprehend anything. In yoga this level of functioning is called kṣipta. A slightly better condition than kṣipta is what is called muḍha. Here the mind is like a dull, sleepy, heavy buffalo. There is hardly any inclination to act, to respond, or to observe. This could be a temporary situation or a more regular affair. There are many reasons for this--overeating, lack of sleep, exhaustion, drugs, or simply an individual's constitution. It can also come about when a person has lost a dear one, has failed to succeed in what he wanted to do, or because of many errors in perception. His attempts to succeed in life have failed and so there is a basic diffidence toward action. Another way the mind functions is called vikṣipta. We act but we have doubts; distractions come about, there are obstacles. The set direction of action does not look right and we don't know what to do about it. The fourth way the mind functions is called ekāgrata. Here clarity has come about and we have direction and are able to proceed. What we want to do is much clearer and distractions hardly matter. This is also called dhāraṇā which was explained earlier. Yoga is actually the beginning of ekāgrata. Yoga suggests means to create conditions that gradually move the kṣipta level of mind towards ekāgrata.

When ekāgrata develops, it culminates in what is called the state of nirodha. This is when the mind and the interest almost become one as if they have merged. For example, had I explained this particular concept to you in the beginning of our studies, I would have had many ideas of approach, references, memories. But as I continue to speak to you more and more my direction of approach to this concept of nirodha becomes set and I hardly need to question it. Now, I am not lost in my explanation nor am I overly conscious about this class to whom I am explaining the concept. I do not worry about your reactions to this or that; to examples I give to make points clear and how I put them into words. In this process my mind has only one interest. It is almost as if my mind is completely enveloped by it. Nothing else bothers me and all my understandings with regard to this concept of nirodha come before me and I am full of it. It follows, therefore, at this moment that nothing other than this subject is before me. This is what the word nirodha means. Rudh represents the envelopment of a particular interest, ni means the intensity of that envelopment. This is a moment the mind functions with no division of activity. The whole mind functions in one area and nothing else can interfere. The word nirodha also means "restraint." It is not by restraining the mind that it will move and become involved in a particular direction of choice. It is the other way round; that is, so strongly and intensely the mind has moved toward one area and has become absorbed in one area that there is no "infiltration." Therefore, nirodha, meaning "restraint," is just an effect of nirodha meaning "complete absorption." "Citta vṛtti nirodha" is how yoga is defined in the Yoga Sūtra. It means that the mind has one and only one activity in all its totality and that the other activities which would distract the mind are absent.

How then do distractions come about? They are there because the mind (citta) has various modes of actions. Through the help of the senses the mind can see or perceive the many things in the world. It can also, on the basis of limited observation, infer the whole. We deduce that it is going to rain when there are dark clouds slowly moving toward us. The mind can also conjure things based simply on words. For example, if I say, "Madras is very pleasant in December," you take it as being that way. For years we have been observing and responding to many things in life and most of the time we are able to recall those observations and responses. This is possible because the mind also has the faculty of retaining something that has been experienced. Added to all of these capabilities it is possible for us to imagine things, and in this, the mind is unlimited. Different actions from the past condition us and block us from seeing things as they are. We already have set ideas about things and we can't get away from them. Examples of this are the notion we have in India that most Americans are rich; or the American idea that all Hindus are vegetarians.

Added to all these capabilities the mind has also inherited a quality of inaction, that is, when we want to do something we don't feel like doing it, or we feel sleepy. The mind has another characteristic. When we want to keep quiet something inside forces us to do what seems like a hundred different things.

It should not be inferred that all of these faculties of the mind, such as observations, inference, memory, imagination, inactivity, hyperactivity, are detrimental. They are necessary to life, but left to itself the mind develops its own way of movement and we end up unable to take full advantage of these faculties. That is why the Yoga Sūtra says that all activities of the mind could be favorable or unfavorable. What we try to do in yoga is simply to create conditions so that the mind becomes a most useful instrument for action. And this can only be done gradually. Any "short-cut method" is an illusion. This gradual procedure may involve a number of intelligent means, all of which come within the realm of yoga sādhana; be it the practice of āsana, the study of the Yoga Sūtra, regulating the breath, complete surrender to Īśvara, detachment in action, visiting a holy man, or investigating the nature of sleep. At different times and for different people different suggestions are necessary. Somehow the mind is brought gradually into a state where it can be completely and intimately involved in a particular understanding or activity. There is little doubt that the clarity that this brings about is total and complete. It is not based on ideas or errors of judgment because the mind at that moment is not elsewhere.

Who does not seek a situation where he is able to understand things clearly, discover new things, and remove or clear away wrong perceptions? If there is one thing that can be said about what happens in the state of nirodha it is this: one sees and one knows. Whatever the mind becomes involved with, it sees completely and knows thoroughly, so much so that there is little left to be known. As we are able to continue with this process, we can see beyond the normal threshold of observation. That is why they say a yogi is a wise man. Not because others cannot see what he has seen but because he has seen something others have not seen, he has seen more than others have seen, and he has seen it ahead of others.

APPENDIX

The following *āsanas* consist of fourteen practice sessions similar to those used by the beginners in the January Special Studies Program. These sequences should not be practiced as exercises in isolation, but in conjunction with knowledge attained either through comprehension of the lectures or, preferably, the direction of a competent teacher.

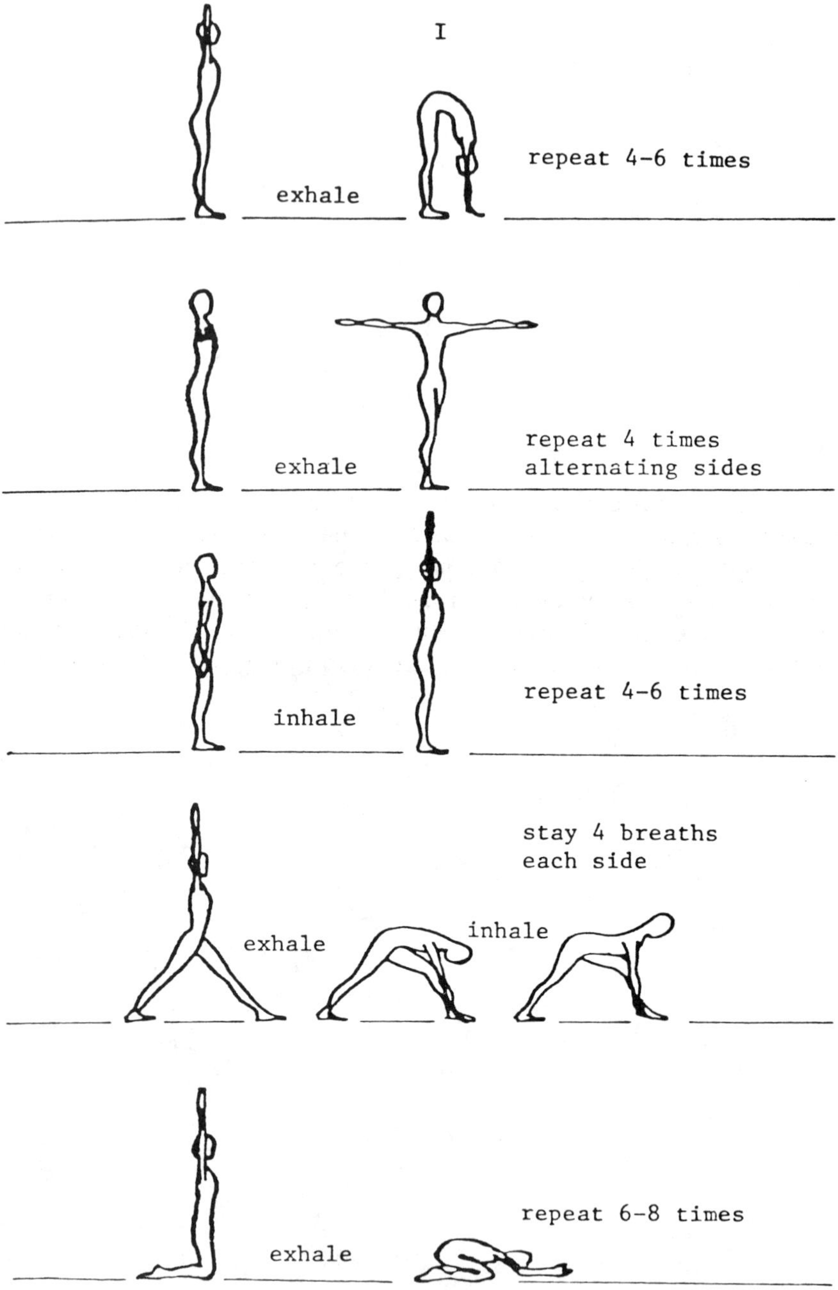
I
repeat 4-6 times
exhale
repeat 4 times
alternating sides
exhale
repeat 4-6 times
inhale
stay 4 breaths
each side
exhale
inhale
repeat 6-8 times
exhale

rest

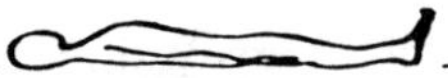

prāṇāyāma: long timed inhalation
pause - free exhalation

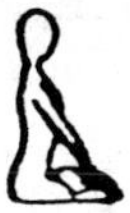

rest

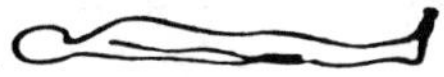

II

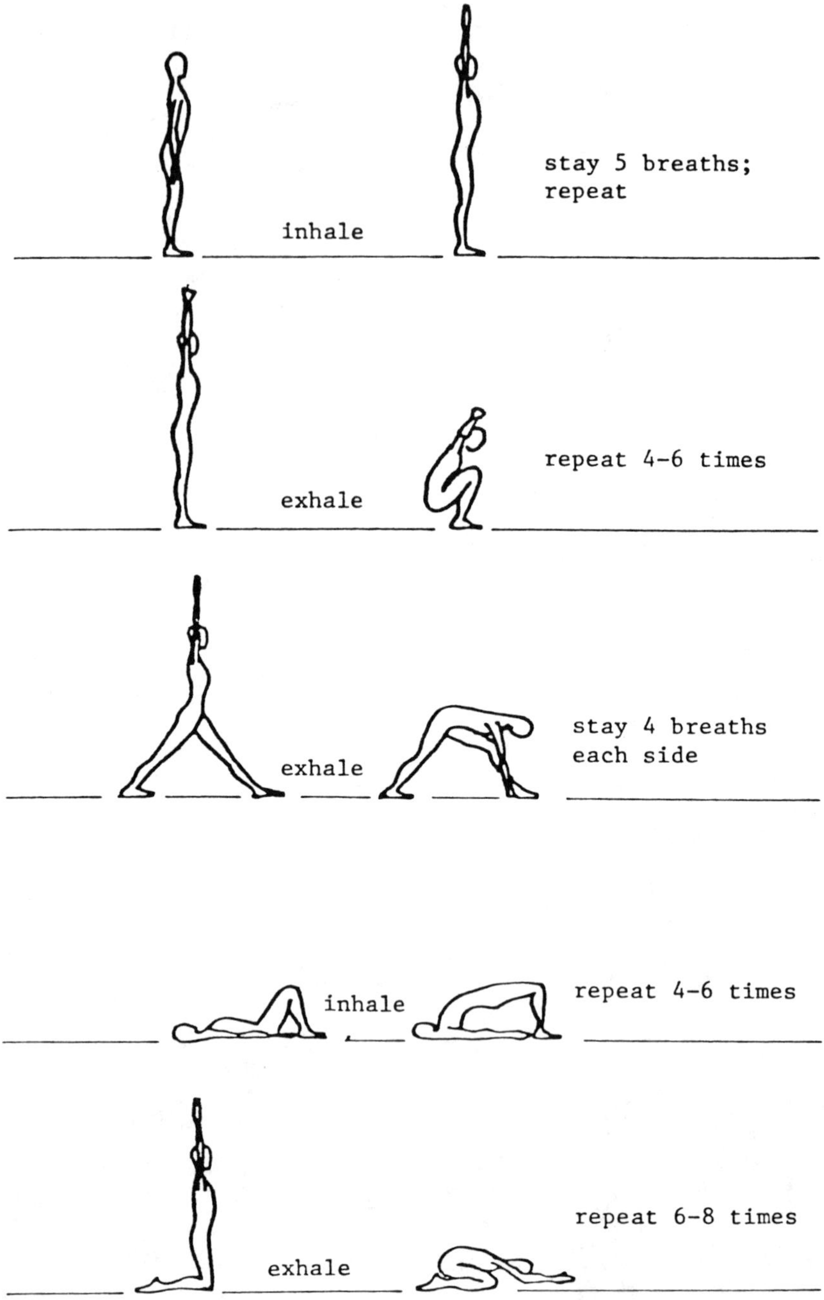
inhale
stay 5 breaths;
repeat
exhale
repeat 4-6 times
exhale
stay 4 breaths
each side
inhale
repeat 4-6 times
exhale
repeat 6-8 times

rest

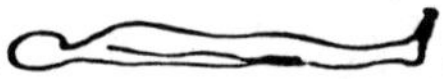

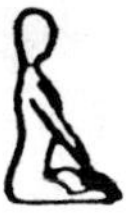

prānāyāma: free inhalation - pause - long timed exhalation

rest

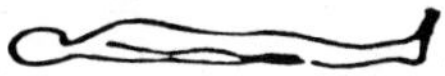

III

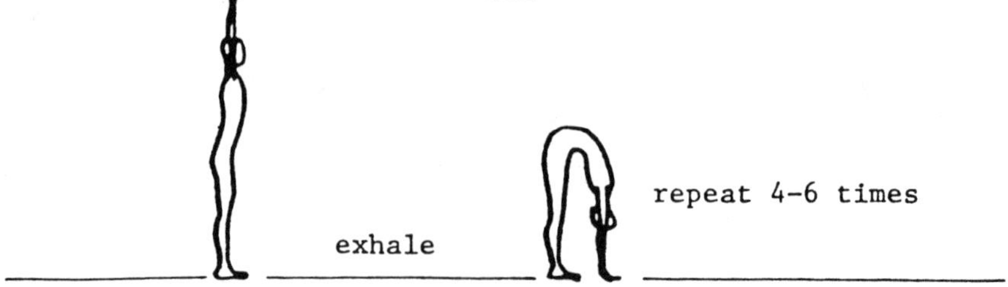
exhale
repeat 4-6 times

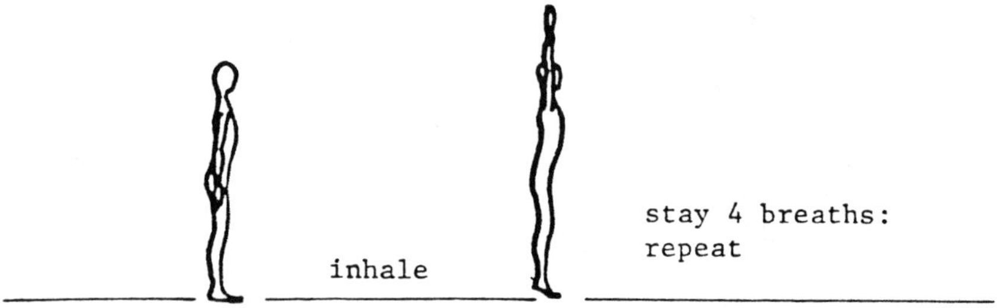
inhale
stay 4 breaths:
repeat

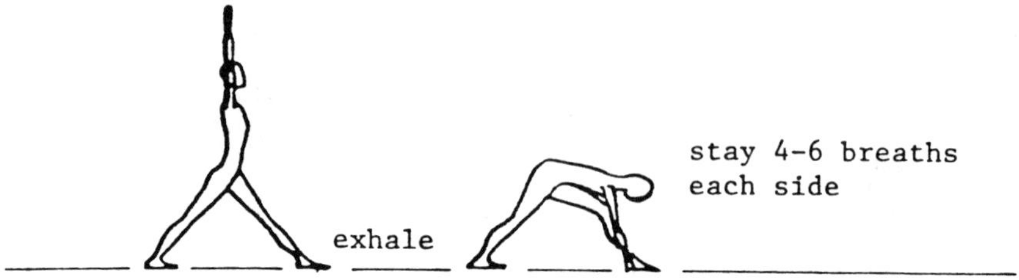
exhale
stay 4-6 breaths
each side

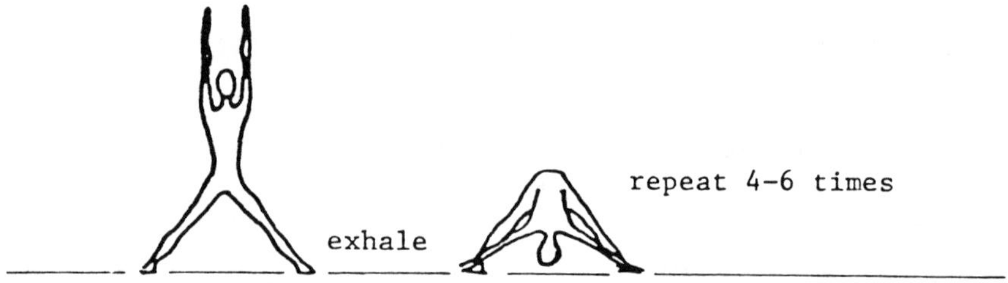
exhale
repeat 4-6 times

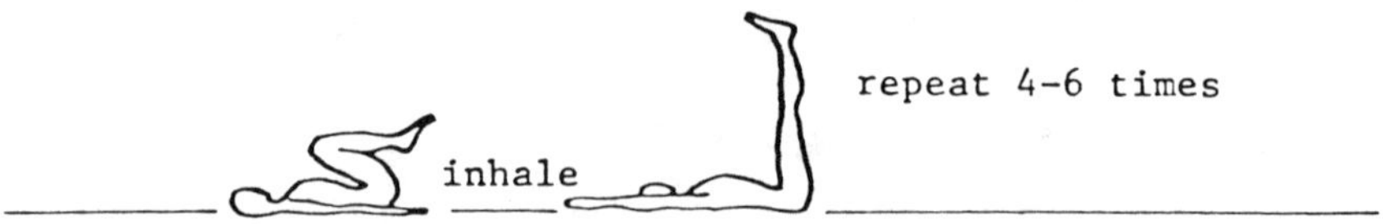
inhale
repeat 4-6 times

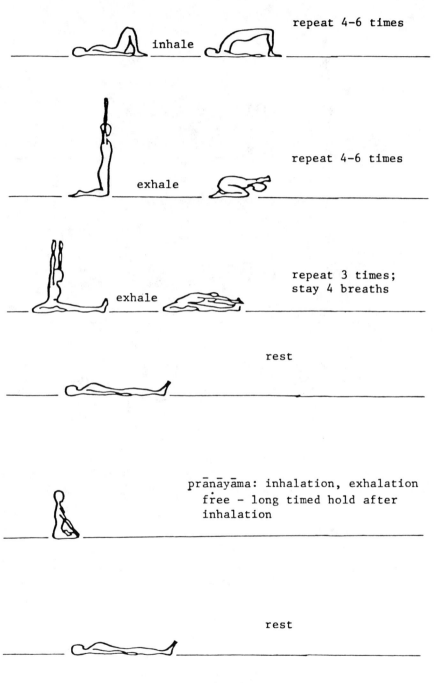

repeat 4-6 times

inhale

repeat 4-6 times

exhale

repeat 3 times;
stay 4 breaths

exhale

rest

prānāyāma: inhalation, exhalation free - long timed hold after inhalation

rest

IV

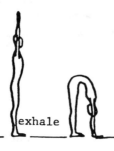

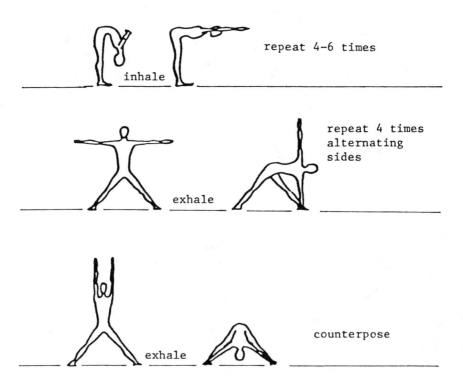

exhale
repeat 2 times;
stay 4-6 breaths
inhale
repeat 4-6 times
exhale
repeat 4 times
alternating
sides
exhale
counterpose

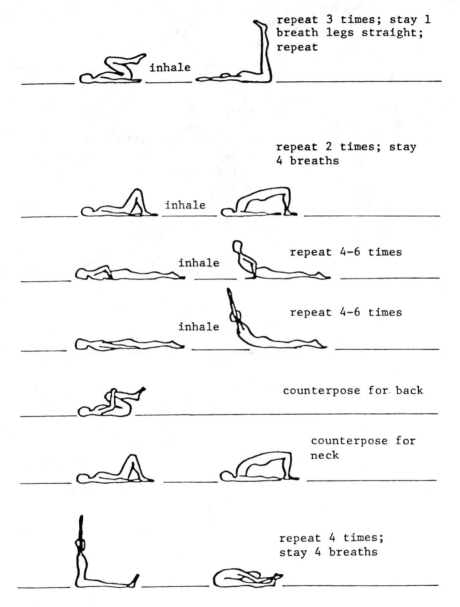

inhale

repeat 3 times; stay 1
breath legs straight;
repeat

repeat 2 times; stay
4 breaths

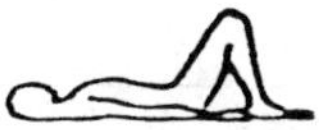

inhale

inhale

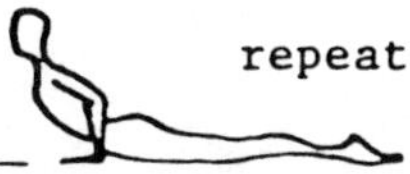

repeat 4-6 times

inhale

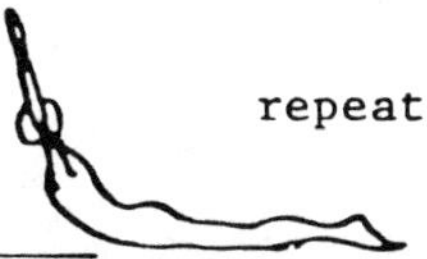

repeat 4-6 times

counterpose for back

counterpose for
neck

repeat 4 times;
stay 4 breaths

rest

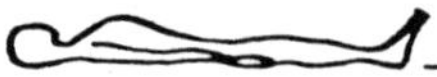

prāṇāyāma: inhalation, exhalation
free - pause - long timed hold
after exhalation

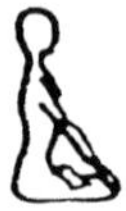

rest

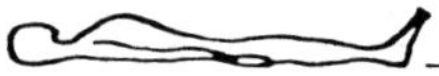

V

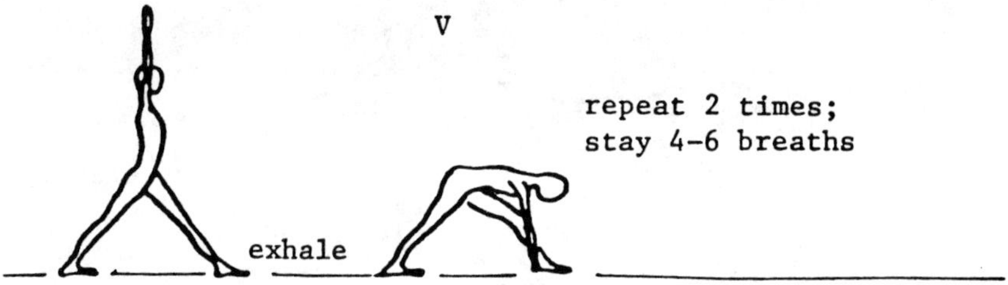
exhale
repeat 2 times;
stay 4-6 breaths

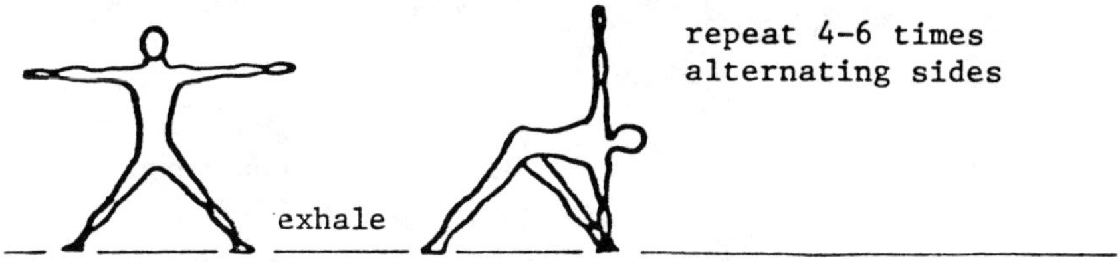
exhale
repeat 4-6 times
alternating sides

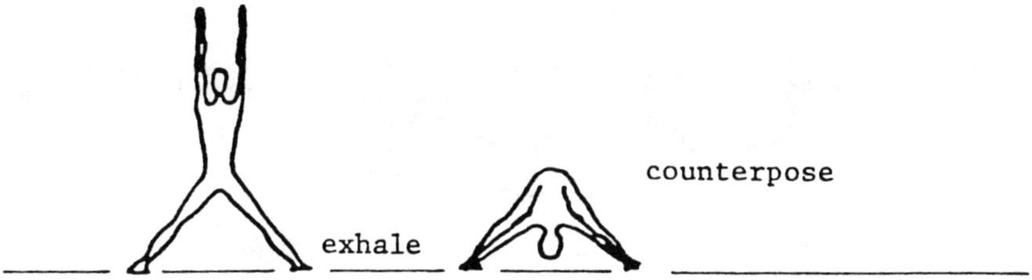
exhale
counterpose

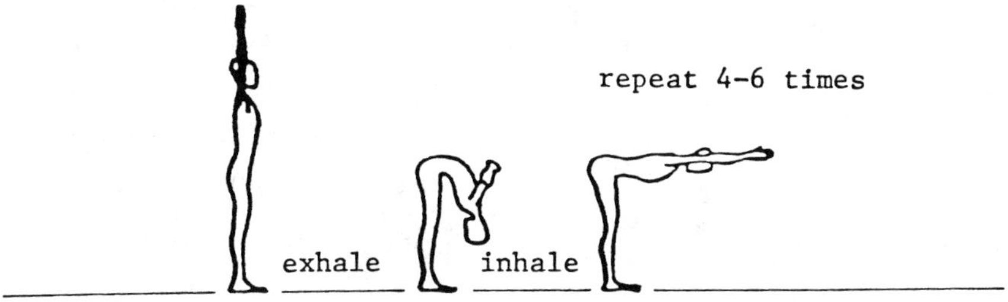
exhale
inhale
repeat 4-6 times

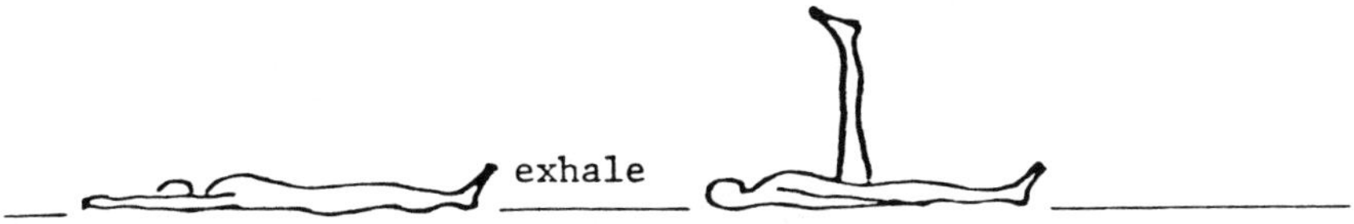
exhale
repeat 4-6 times
alternating legs

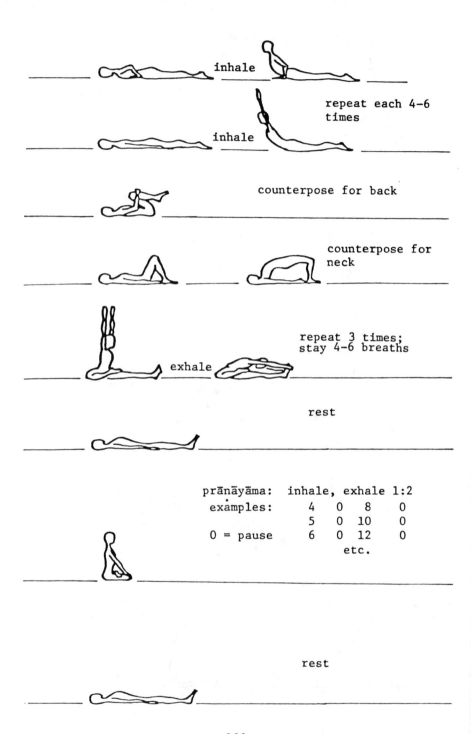

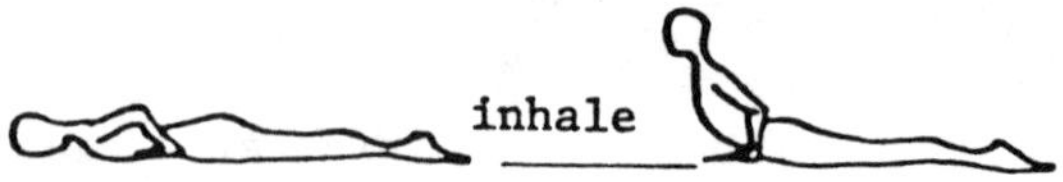

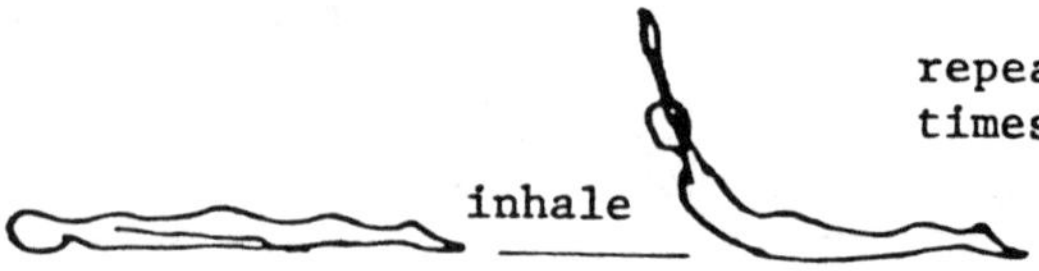

repeat each 4-6 times

counterpose for back

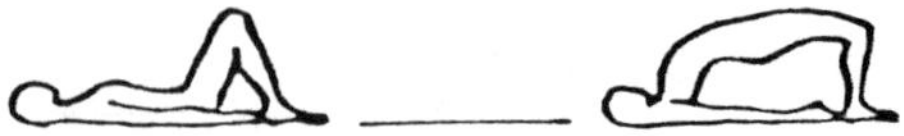

counterpose for neck

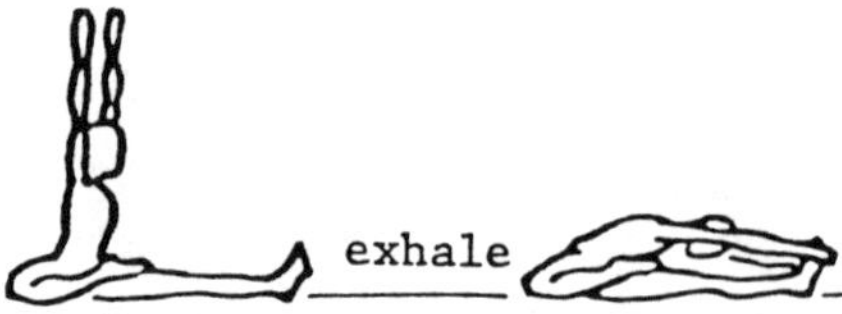

repeat 3 times; stay 4-6 breaths

rest

prāṇāyāma:	inhale, exhale 1:2				
examples:		4	0	8	0
		5	0	10	0
0 = pause		6	0	12	0
			etc.		

rest

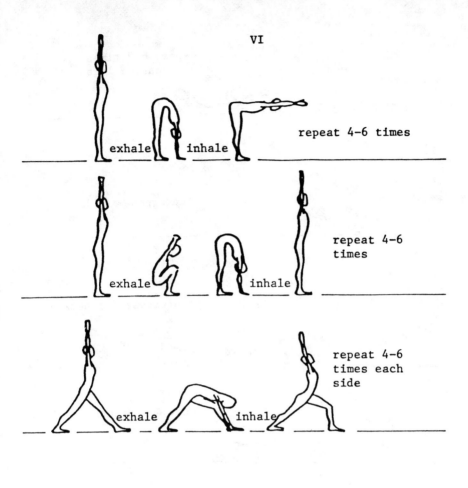

VI

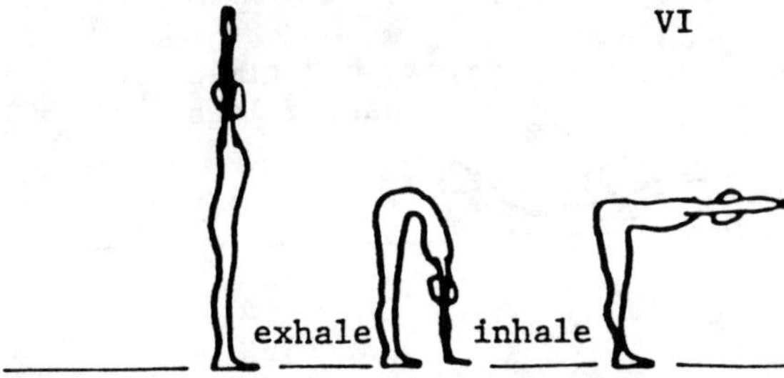

repeat 4-6 times

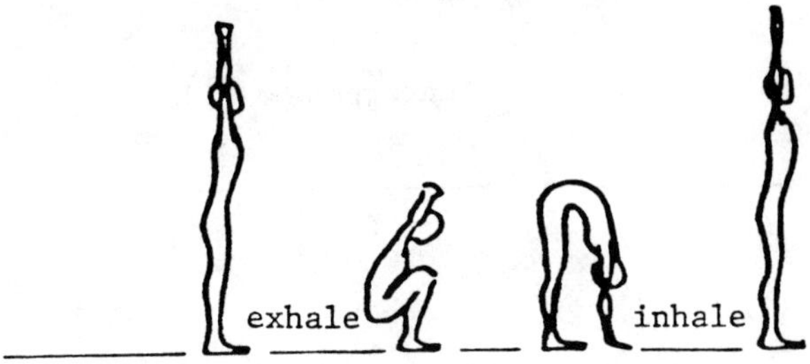

repeat 4-6 times

repeat 4-6 times each side

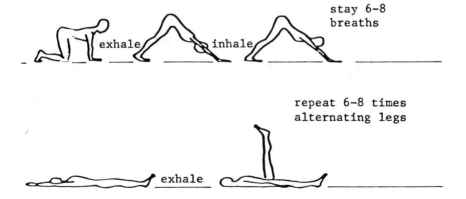

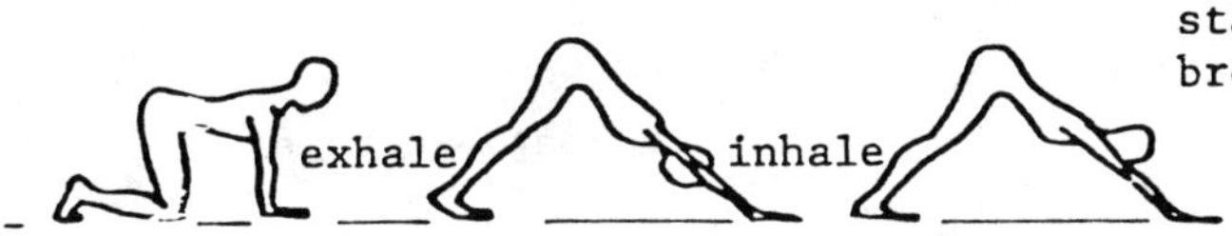

stay 6-8 breaths

repeat 6-8 times alternating legs

repeat 6-8 times
alternating legs

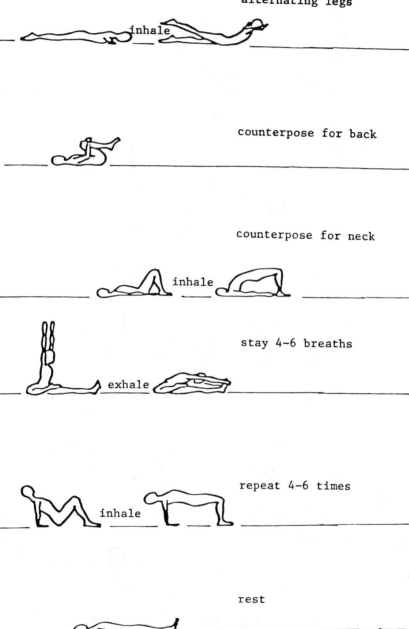

counterpose for back

counterpose for neck

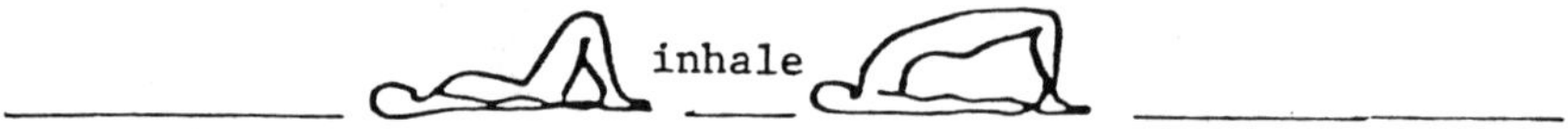

stay 4-6 breaths

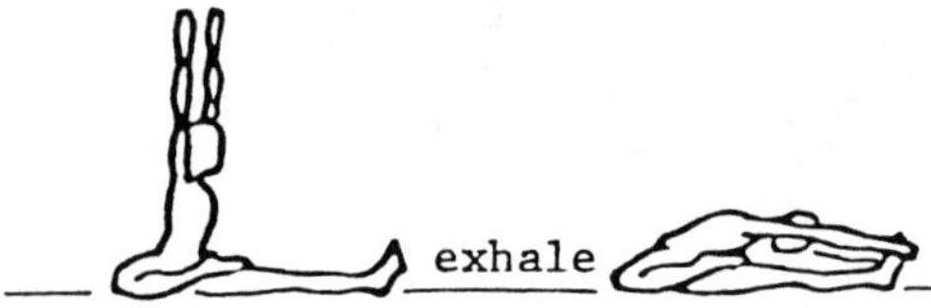

repeat 4-6 times

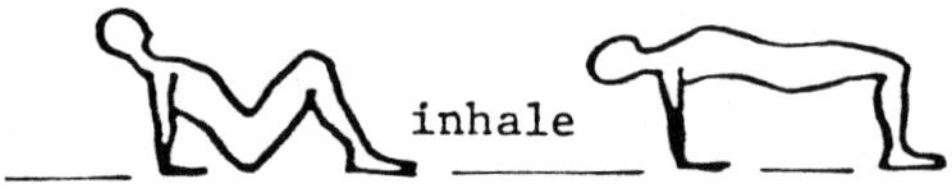

rest

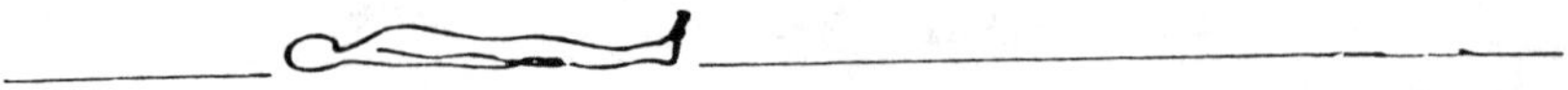

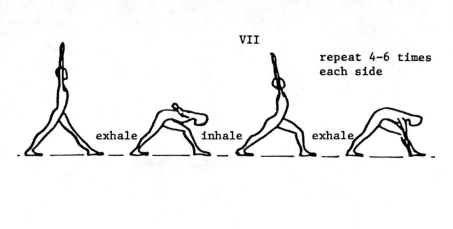

VII

repeat 4-6 times
each side

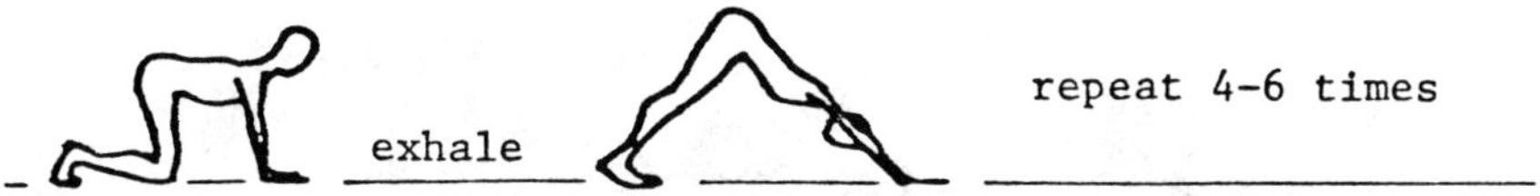

repeat 4-6 times

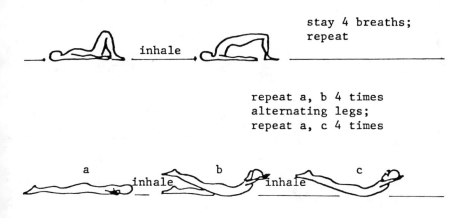

stay 4 breaths;
repeat

repeat a, b 4 times
alternating legs;
repeat a, c 4 times

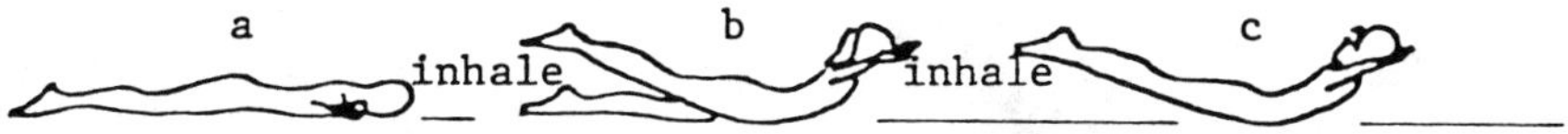

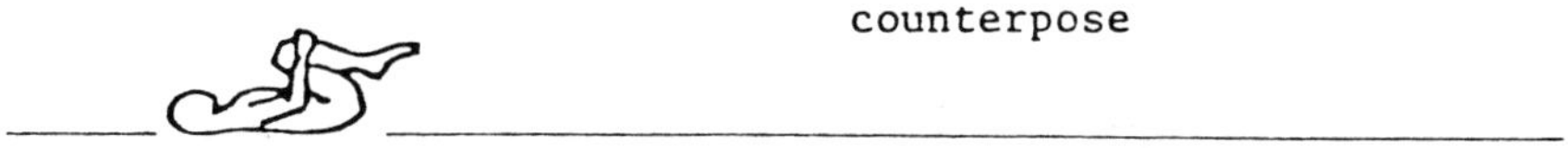

counterpose

repeat 4 times;
stay 4 breaths

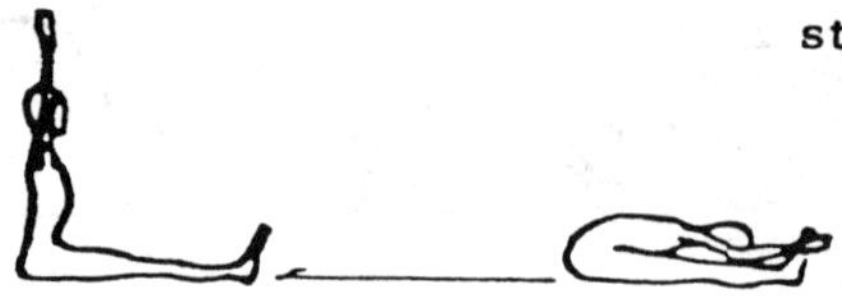

repeat 4 times

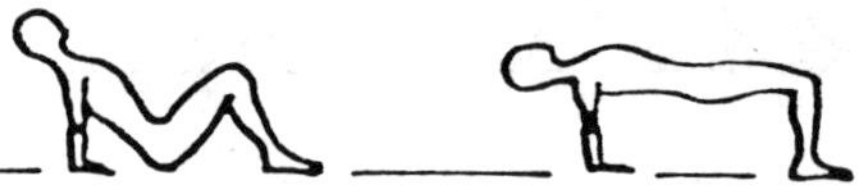

rest

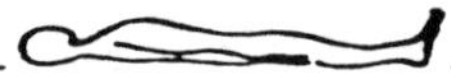

prāṇāyāma:	inhale, exhale 1:2				
examples		4	0	8	0
		5	0	10	0
		6	0	12	0
			etc.		

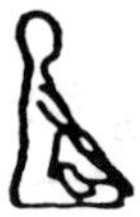

rest

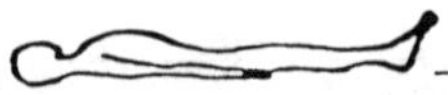

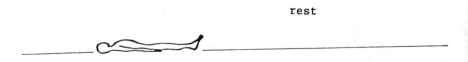

VIII. Plan a course with 8 of the following postures, using a maximum of 100 breaths.

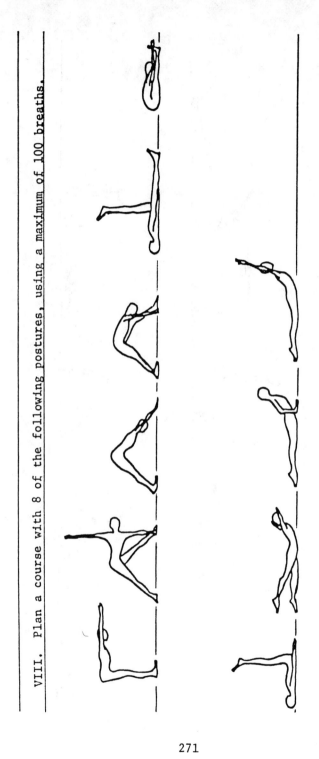

IX. Plan a course with 6 of the following postures, including the first two.

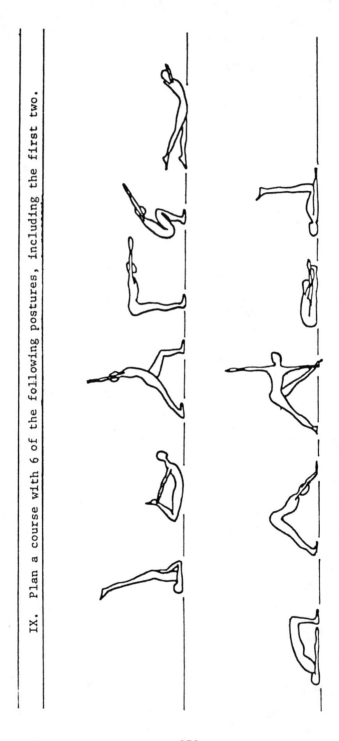

X

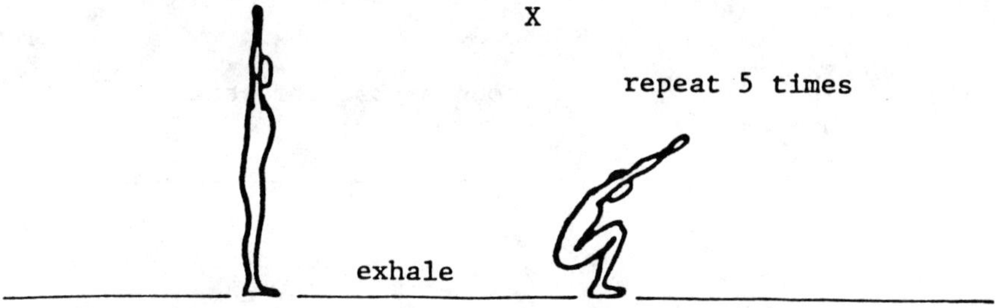
repeat 5 times
exhale

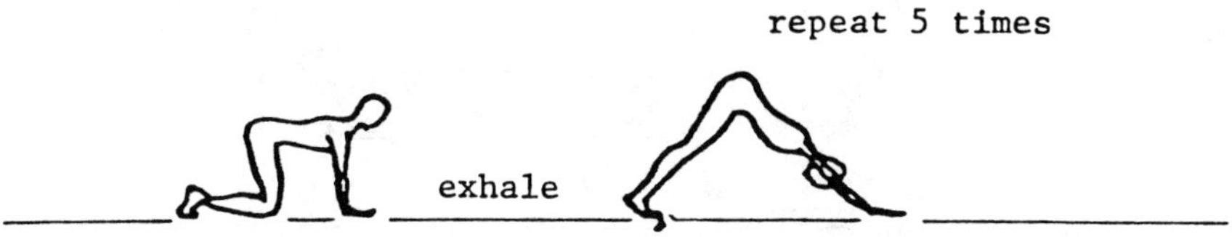
repeat 5 times
exhale

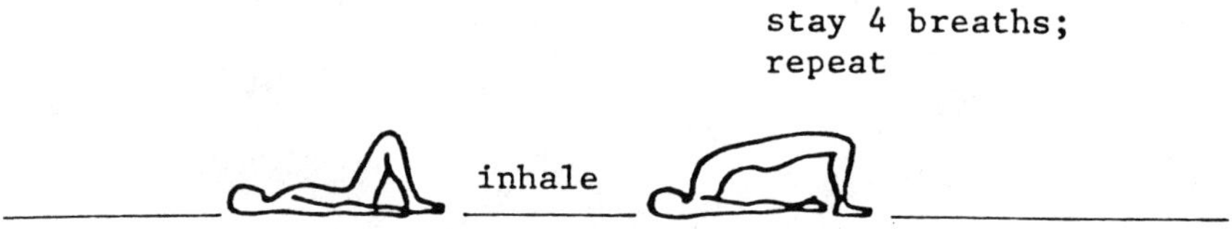
stay 4 breaths;
repeat
inhale

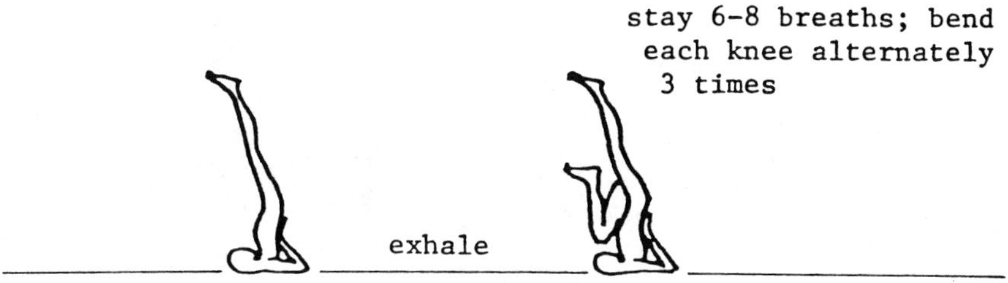
stay 6-8 breaths; bend
each knee alternately
3 times
exhale

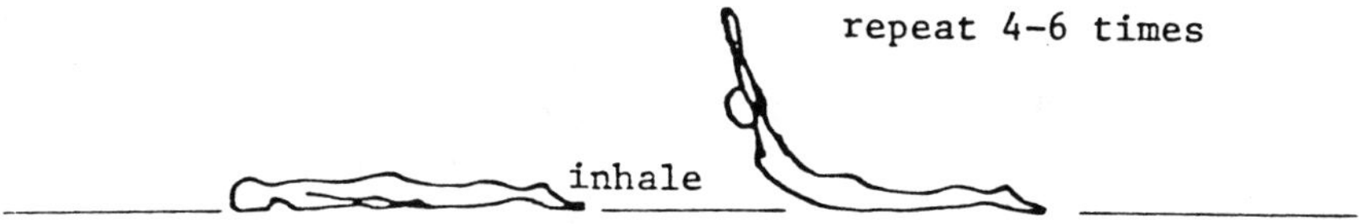
repeat 4-6 times
inhale

counterpose for back

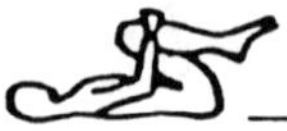

counterpose
for neck

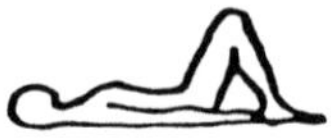

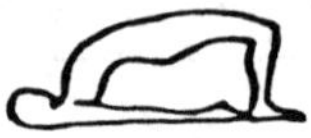

rest

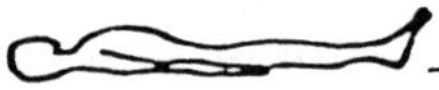

XI

repeat 4-6 times
each side

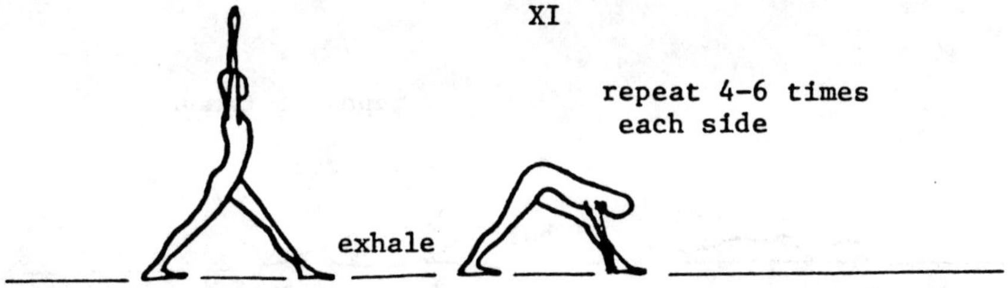

repeat 4-6 times

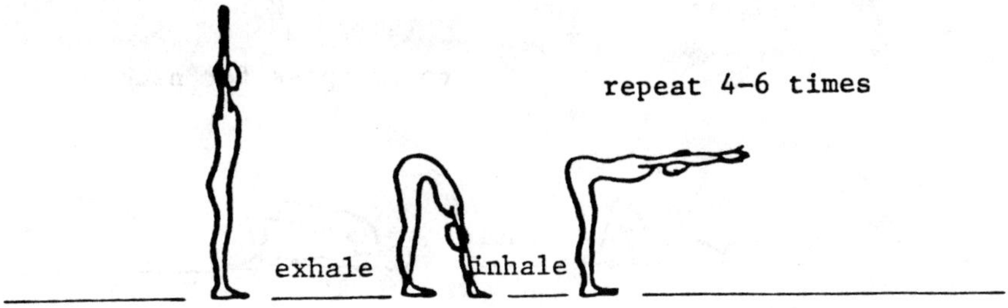

repeat 4-6 times

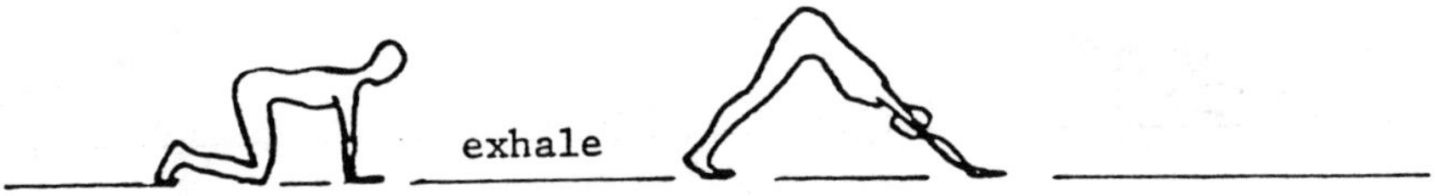

stay 4 breaths;
repeat

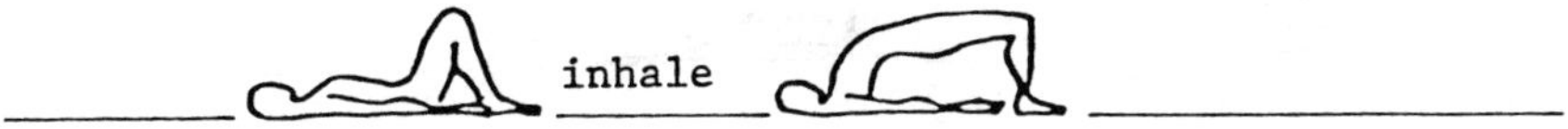

stay 8-12 breaths; bend each
leg alternately 3 times

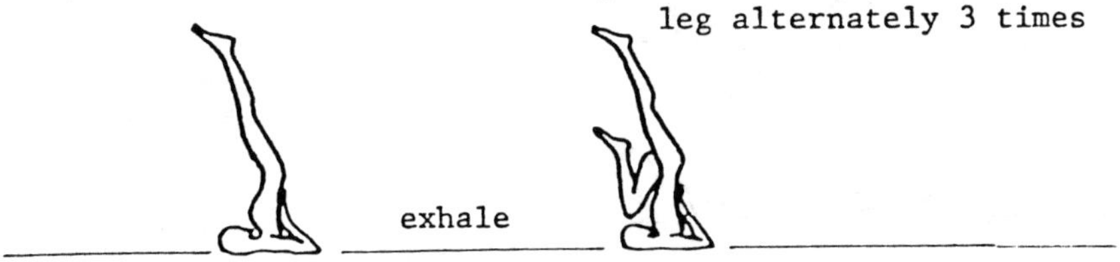

repeat 6 times

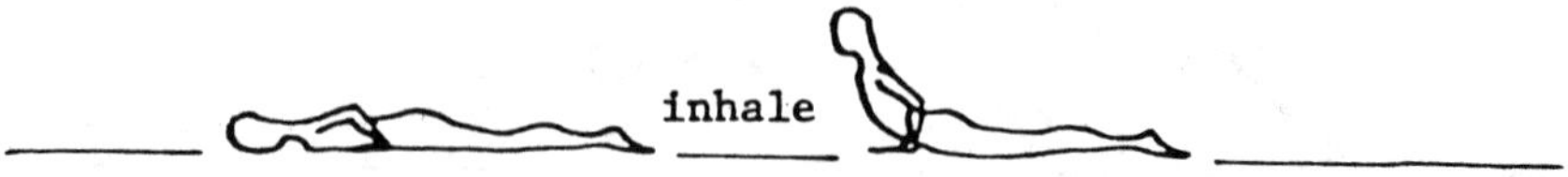

counterpose for neck

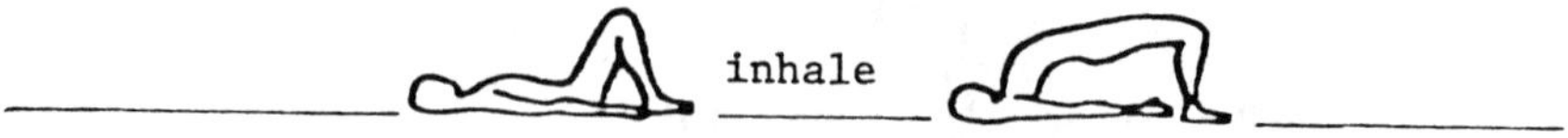

counterpose for back

repeat 6 times

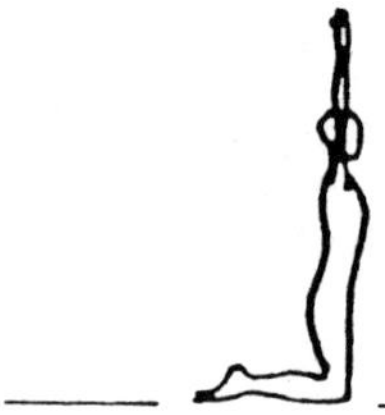

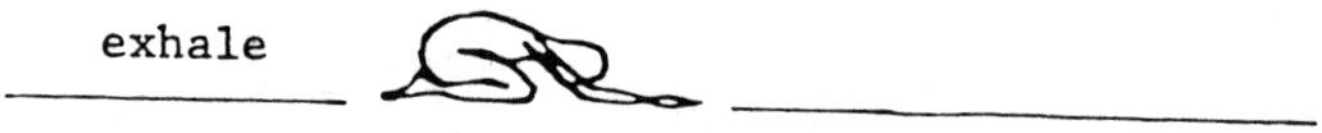

rest

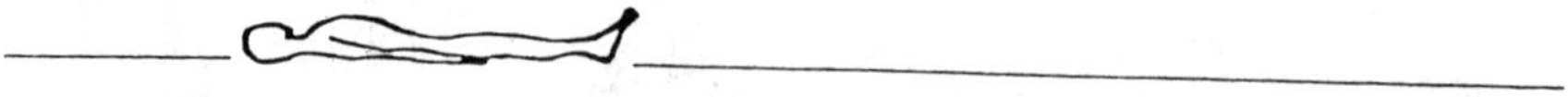

XII
Preparation for Shoulderstand

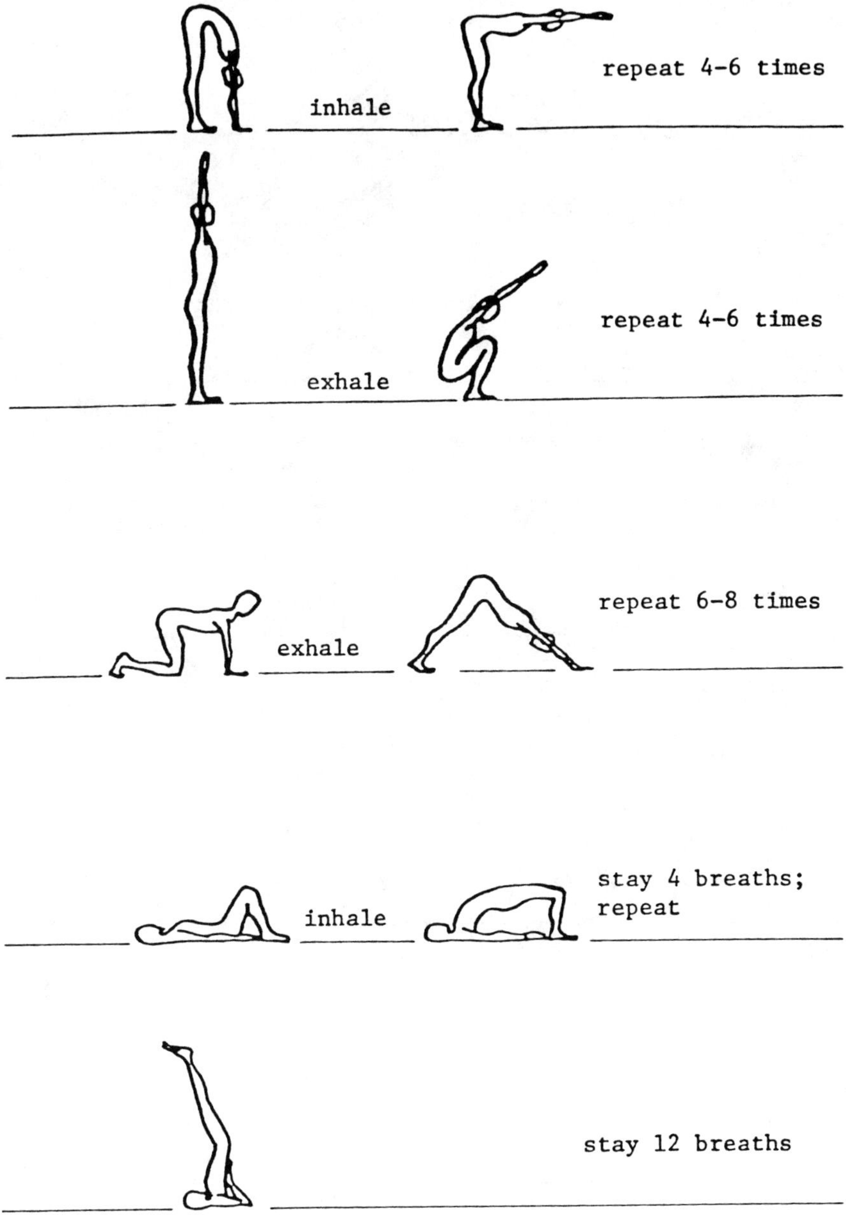

counterpose for shoulderstand -
repeat 4-6 times

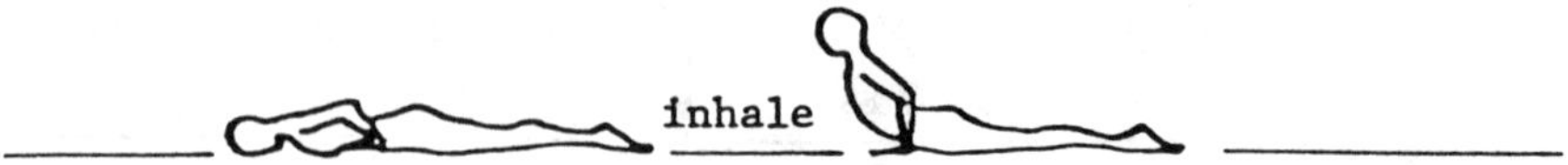

counterpose for back

counterpose for
neck

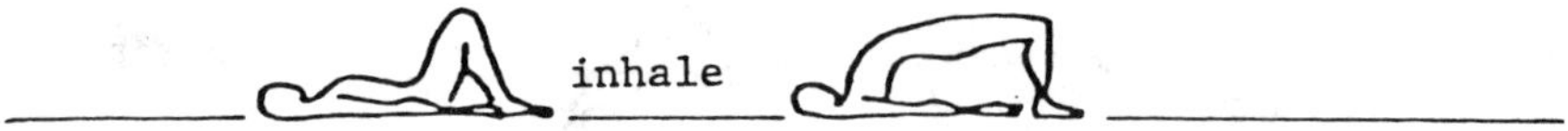

repeat 6 times

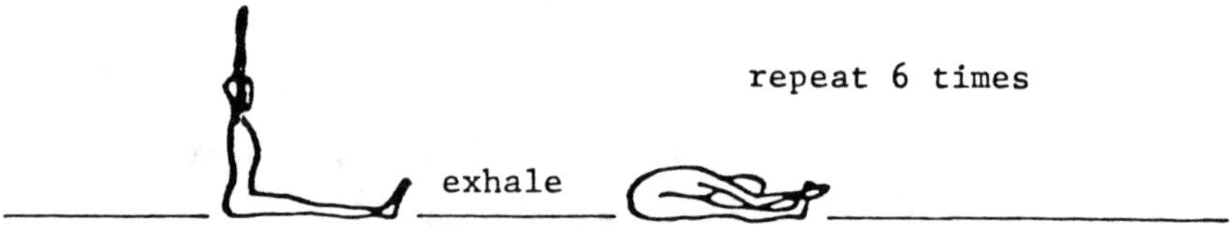

rest

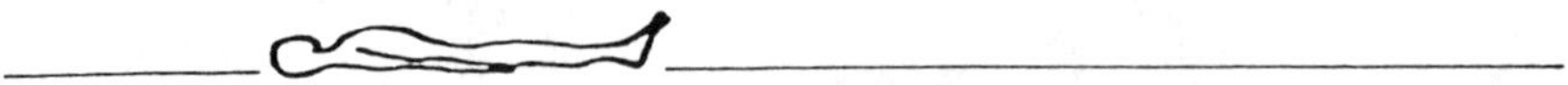

XIII
Preparation for Headstand

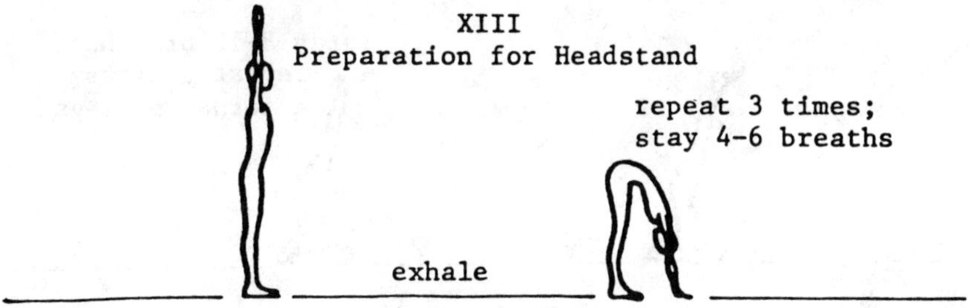

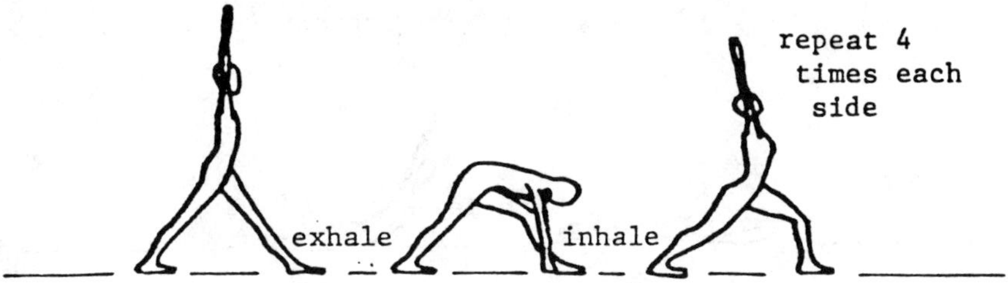

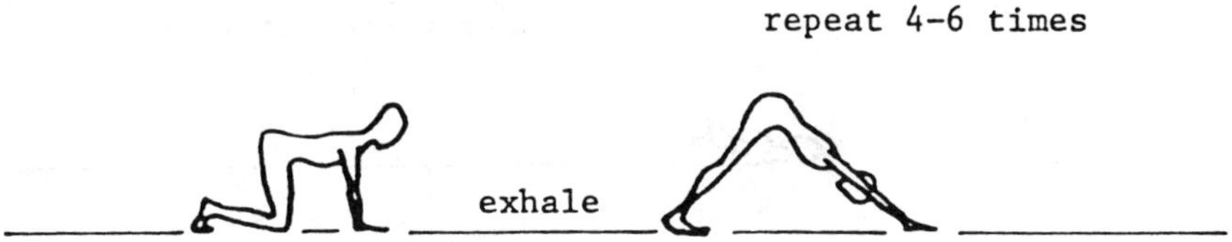

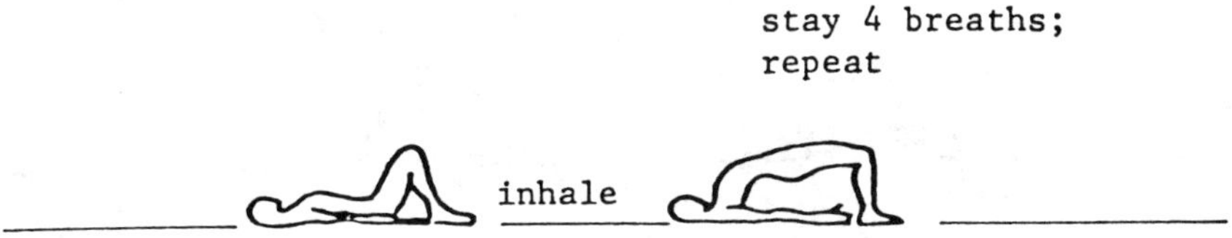

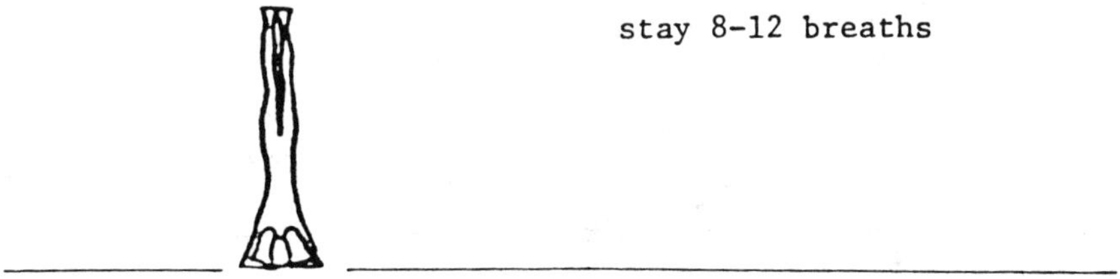

stay 8-12 breaths;
repeat 3 times
alternating legs

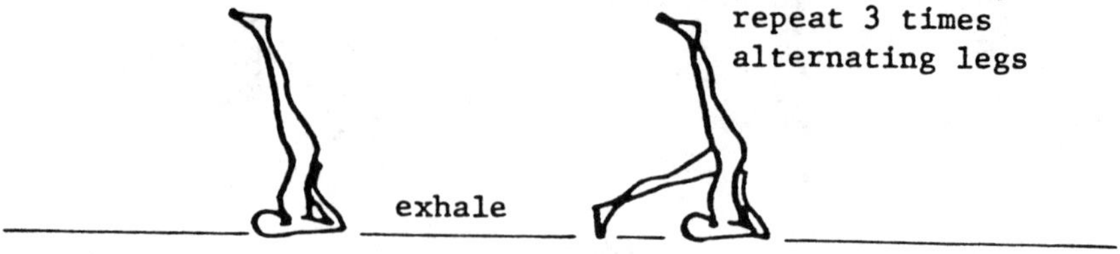

repeat 4-6 times

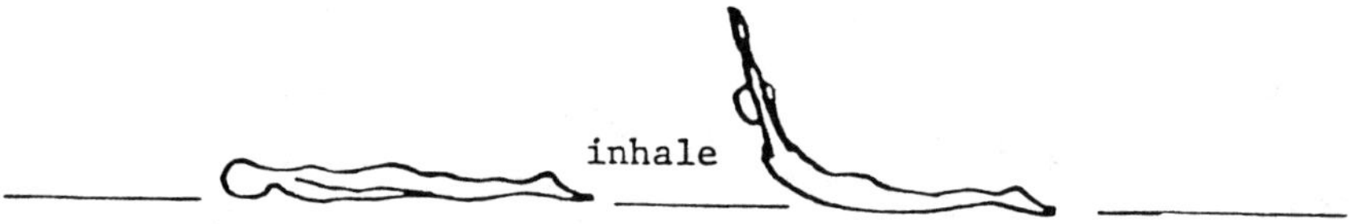

counterpose for back

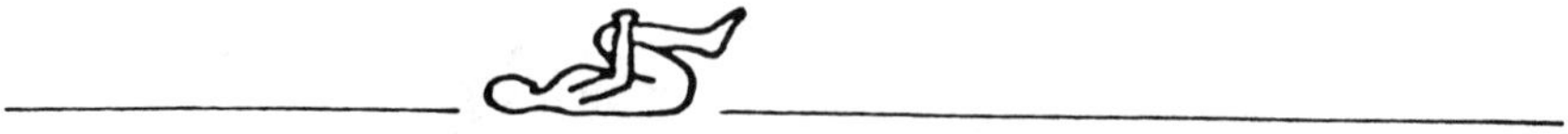

counterpose
for neck

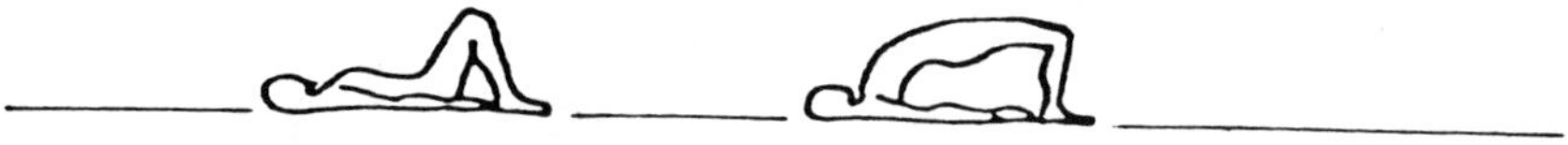

rest

prāṇāyāma: inhale, exhale 1:2

See Course VII

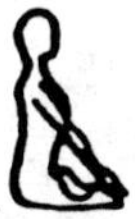

rest

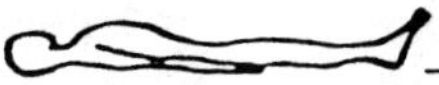

XIV
Preparation for Prāṇāyāma

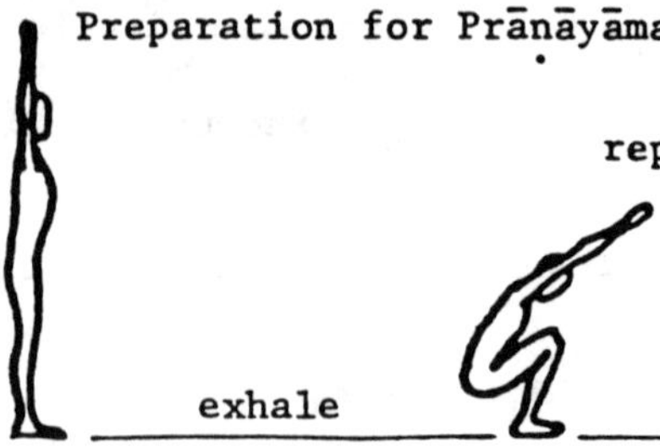

repeat 4-6 times

exhale

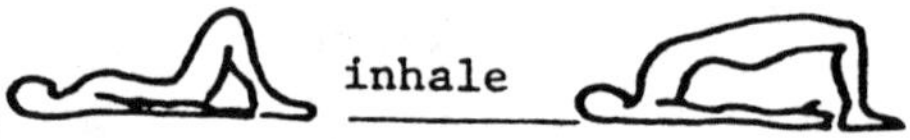

stay 4 breaths;
repeat

inhale

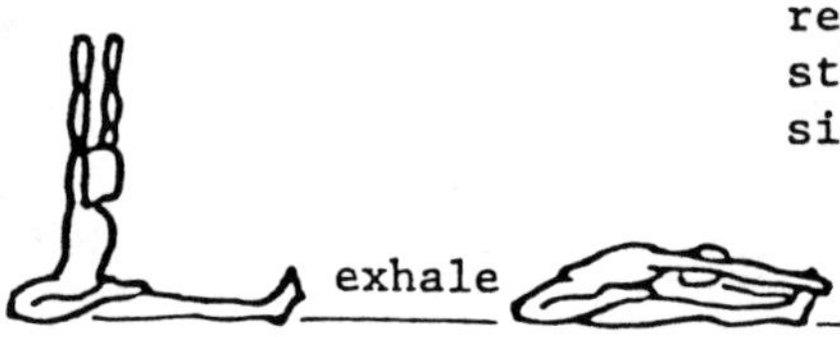

repeat 3 times;
stay 4 breaths each
side

exhale

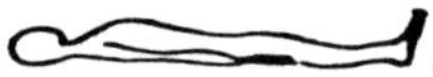

rest

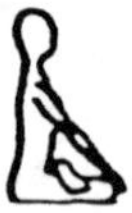

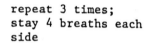

prāṇāyāma:

	inhale	hold	exhale	hold	breaths
	5	0	10	0	6
example	5	5	10	0	6
	5	5	10	5	6
	5	0	10	0	6

rest

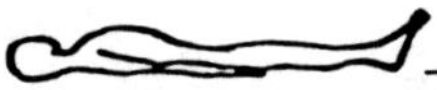

SELECTED BIBLIOGRAPHY

The Bhagavadgītā. Of numerous translations, one might consult the translation by S. Radhakrishnan. New York: Harper and Row, 1975.

The Gheraṇḍa Saṃhitā. Translated by Rai Bahadur Śrī Chandra Vasu. Delhi: Oriental Books Reprint Corporation, 2nd edition, 1975.

Haṭhapradīpikā of Svātmārāma. Edited by Swami Digambarji and Pt. Raghunathashastri Kokaje. Lonavla, Poona district, India: Kaivalyadhama, S. M. Y. M. Samiti, 1970.

Krishnamacharya, T. Yoga Makaranda. (in Kannada) Mysore, 1934.

__________. Yogāñjali. (in Kannada) Mysore: 2 volumes, 1952.

__________. Yoga Rahasya: Yogi Nathamuni. An unpublished manuscript recording the dictation of T. Krishnamacharya.

__________. Yogāsanagalu. (in Kannada) Mysore: Mysore University, 1973.

Yoga Philosophy of Patañjali. By Swāmi Hariharānanda Araṇya, translated by P. N. Mukerji. Calcutta: University of Calcutta Press, 1977.

Yoga Yajñavalkya. Translated by Sri Prabhad C. Divanji. Journal of the Bombay Branch of the Royal Asiatic Society. Reprint, Monograph No. 3, 1954.

INDEX OF FIGURES

GENERAL INDEX

Editors' Note: Yoga as a personal practice and process in the human heritage has a technical Sanskrit vocabulary developed in India. Most of the technical terms, so rich in connotation and nuance, have not yet found their adequate English counterpart. We recommend that one become familiar with these terms, the most important of which are noted in this index. See also Index of Figures, pp. 287-292.

time of day for practice.
See under practice, planning of
udāna-vāyu, 143
udāra, 184-185
uḍḍīyana bandha, 195, 197-199
upādāna kāraṇa, 226
Upaniṣads, 216, 249
upaviṣṭha koṇāsana, 49
uṣṭrāsana, 133
uttānāsana, 51, 62, 92, 101
utkaṭāsana, 51, 67, 99
vajrāsana, 204-205
vāyu, 246
Veda, 1
vicāra, 161
vicchina, 184
vikalpa, 71
vikṣipta, 251
viloma krama prāṇāyāma, 168
viloma ujjāyī prāṇāyāma, 121
vinyāsa, 49, 113
viparyaya, 71
vīrāsana, 204-205
vīrya, 110
viṣamavṛtti prāṇāyāma, 121
viśeṣa, 211
viśeṣa puruṣa, 211
Viṣṇu, 217
vitarka, 161
viveka, 74
viveki, 69
yama, 107 ff., 133, 146-148, 152, 218, 231
yoga, meaning of, purpose of, and practice of 1-254 passim
yoga sādhana, 253
Yoga Sūtra, 1-254 passim
yogi, 254
Zen, 231-233